A Virtue-Based Defense
of Perinatal Hospice

Aaron Cobb's book makes a twofold contribution: to our understanding of the value and virtues of perinatal hospice, and to contemporary moral theory. His personal experience as a father and professional vocation as a philosopher together provide uncommon insight.

—*Bernard Prusak, King's College (PA), USA*

Aaron Cobb's *A Virtue-Based Defense of Perinatal Hospice* is a fascinating book. His examination of perinatal palliative and hospice care is excellent. His appropriation of virtue ethics and the notions of exemplary persons and communities, as well as his focus on the needs of the entire family, are very helpful. The book deals with a variety of important moral and existential issues that arise in such situations, and in light of its approach to them it deserves both a wide reading and widespread reflective application.

—*Michael W. Austin, Eastern Kentucky University, USA*

Perinatal hospice is a novel form of care for an unborn child who has been diagnosed with a significantly life-limiting condition. In this book, Aaron D. Cobb develops a virtue-based defense of the value of perinatal hospice. He characterizes its promotion and provision as a common project of individuals, local communities, and institutions working together to provide exemplary care. Engaging with important themes from the work of Alasdair MacIntyre and Robert Adams, he shows how perinatal hospice manifests virtues crucial to meeting the needs of families in these difficult circumstances. As a work of applied virtue ethics, this book has important normative, social, and political implications for the creation and development of structured programs of care. It grounds the view that communities ought (i) to devote resources to ensure that these programs are widely available and (ii) to develop social structures that promote awareness of and accessibility to these forms of care. *A Virtue-Based Defense of Perinatal Hospice* will be of interest to philosophers working in bioethics and applied virtue ethics, as well as scholars in the fields of neonatology, nursing, palliative and hospice care, and counseling who are interested in the study of perinatal hospice.

Aaron D. Cobb is an associate professor of philosophy at Auburn University at Montgomery. His recent scholarship has focused on moral and intellectual virtues. He is the author of *Loving Samuel: Suffering, Dependence, and the Calling of Love*, a philosophical and theological memoir on the life and death of his son.

Routledge Annals of Bioethics

Series Editors:
Mark J. Cherry
St. Edward's University, USA
Ana Smith Iltis
Saint Louis University, USA

For more information about this series, please visit: www.routledge.com/Routledge-Annals-of-Bioethics/book-series/RAB

A Virtue-Based Defense of Perinatal Hospice

Aaron D. Cobb

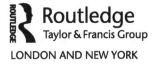

Routledge
Taylor & Francis Group

LONDON AND NEW YORK

First published 2020 by Routledge

2 Park Square, Milton Park, Abingdon, Oxon OX14 4RN
605 Third Avenue, New York, NY 10017

Routledge is an imprint of the Taylor & Francis Group, an informa business

First issued in paperback 2021

Publisher's Note

The publisher has gone to great lengths to ensure the quality of this reprint
but points out that some imperfections in the original copies may be apparent.

Library of Congress Cataloging-in-Publication Data
A catalog record for this book has been requested

ISBN: 978-0-8153-7299-8 (hbk)
ISBN: 978-1-03-217758-8 (pbk)
DOI: 10.4324/9781351244473

Typeset in Sabon
by Apex CoVantage, LLC

To Alisha, Micah, and Samuel

Contents

Acknowledgments

In his work, *Dependent Rational Animals: Why Human Beings Need the Virtues*, Alasdair MacIntyre writes, "generally and characteristically, what and how far we are able to give depends in part on what and how far we received" (99). Given my indebtedness to MacIntyre's work, it is fitting to recognize those whose generosity made it possible for me to complete this project.

I am indebted to my colleagues at Auburn University at Montgomery for their encouragement in my scholarly efforts. I am especially grateful to Michael Burger, Bob Evans, Darren Harris-Fain, Eric Sterling, and Tara Woods for their support on this project. Many of my friends and colleagues offered constructive feedback on this work. In my initial published work on perinatal hospice, Craig Boyd, Jeff Hammond, Adam MacLeod, Robert McFarland, Gilbert Meilaender, Philip Reed, and Victoria Seed offered constructive feedback. Mike Austin, Rebecca Konyndyk DeYoung, and Kevin Timpe offered helpful comments on early drafts of the book proposal. Craig Boyd, Gregory Poore, and Bernard Prusak offered extensive comments on the entire manuscript. At various stages in my research for this book, I benefitted greatly from conversations with Ryan Byerly, Patrick Clark, Nathan King, Adam Pelser, and Ryan West.

I am grateful to Kelly Jolley and James Loxley Compton for their invitation to present an early version of Chapter 4 at Auburn University's Philosophy of Religion Workshop. I also benefitted from feedback I received at King's College (Pennsylvania) where I delivered the 2018 *Donald J. Grimes Lecture*. I am especially grateful to Bernard Prusak and Regan Reitsma for their invitation to present this lecture. The students in the King's College Honors Program along with the members of the audience helped me to frame the central chapters of the manuscript. Finally, I am grateful to Jim Delaney for the invitation to present a paper at the 2018 *Ostapenko Center for Ethics in Medicine and Health Care Symposium* at Niagara University. Jim and the other participants in the workshop— Jason Eberl, David Hershenov, Philip Reed, Christopher Tollefesen, and

Patrick Tully—helped me to think through some of the implications of the basic framework I develop in this manuscript.

Work on this project was made possible through the support of a grant from The Beacon Project at Wake Forest University and the Templeton Religion Trust. The opinions expressed in this publication are those of the author and do not necessarily reflect the views of The Beacon Project, Wake Forest University, or the Templeton Religion Trust. I am grateful to William Fleeson, Christian Miller, R. Michael Furr, and Angela Knobel for their work directing this project.

I owe Andrew Weckenmann, Allie Simmons, Mark Cherry, Ana Iltis, and the entire team at Routledge Press a debt of gratitude for the opportunity to write this book. I'm grateful for their work in helping me bring it to press.

Chapters 1, 2, 4, 5, and 7 quote passages from my essay "Acknowledged Dependence and the Virtues of Perinatal Hospice." *Journal of Medicine and Philosophy* 41 (1): 25–40. Chapter 6 includes some revised material from my essay "Compassion and Consolation," in *The Moral Psychology of Compassion*, edited by Justin Caouette and Carolyn Price, 49–60. Rowman & Littlefield. All of this material is used with permission.

I would be remiss if I did not conclude with some personal words of gratitude. Most importantly, I would like to thank my wife, Alisha, and my son, Micah, both of whom offered significant grace and encouragement throughout the time I was writing this book. This small word of thanks is an insufficient expression of my gratitude and love. I am also grateful for the countless ways my life has been enriched by my son Samuel. Writing this book has provided countless opportunities to remember him. I hope that the words of the book adequately convey my ongoing love. I am also grateful for our extended family and friends who continue to love and support us. We are thankful for the ways they help to keep Sam's memory alive. Finally, I need to express thanks to the healthcare providers who cared for my family. I am grateful to Jennifer Logan, MD; Aaron Millage, MD; Erin Jones, NNP; and the excellent nurses in the neonatal intensive care unit including Tina Blankenship, Kasey Emmons, Stacy Hall, Rachel Rascoe, and Jennifer Todd.

1   Toward a Virtue-Based Defense of Perinatal Hospice

I. Introduction

The routine use of ultrasound technology coupled with advances in pre-natal screening have increased diagnostic capacities to detect rare and often significantly life-limiting conditions.[1] These developments raise troubling questions for prospective parents. What should families do if these tests reveal genetic anomalies and congenital defects? Should they terminate the pregnancy in the hope of preventing suffering?[2] If they choose to continue the pregnancy, are they prepared for the potential physical, psychological, emotional, and financial burdens of caring for a child with profound needs? Typically, parents are forced to ask these questions at advanced stages of a wanted pregnancy, reflecting on their options in the shock that follows a devastating diagnosis. Any choice in this context is fraught with difficulty.

Consider a hypothetical case. Jason and his wife Kelly were expect-ing their first child. During the course of Kelly's routine twenty-week ultrasound, their obstetrician detected a number of signs indicative of trisomy 18, a rare chromosomal abnormality in which the child inherits an extra copy of the eighteenth chromosome.[3] This extra genetic material disrupts normal development, giving rise to a range of associated anoma-lies including heart and kidney malformations, abdominal wall defects, and decreased birth size.[4] Children with trisomy 18 often die *in utero*; for those born alive, around 90% will die before their first birthday. Often, children born with this condition measure their lives in the space of hours or days.[5]

Jason and Kelly's obstetrician referred them to a specialist for addi-tional testing. The fetal-maternal health specialist informed them that an amniocentesis could confirm a trisomy 18 diagnosis, providing useful information concerning their choice options. But she noted that there are a limited range of options for children with trisomy 18. Given the prog-nosis, most families choose to interrupt the pregnancy. Whatever their decision, Jason and Kelly needed to choose quickly so that they could pursue the full range of legal options available to them. After relaying this information, the physician left the room to give them a few minutes to consider the options they wished to pursue.

Jason and Kelly loved their daughter; they had been eagerly anticipating her arrival. But the prospect of seeing her suffer was almost unthinkable. How could they endure the remainder of the pregnancy knowing that their daughter would suffer? What was the point if she would die soon after birth? Terminating the pregnancy would prevent her from experiencing pointless pain. It would keep them from having to experience the sorrow of watching her die. After several minutes of silence, Kelly said to Jason, "If the test confirms trisomy 18, I think we need to terminate the pregnancy. I can't imagine continuing under these conditions; the physician said the condition is lethal." Jason agreed, responding, "Either way, she is going to die. At least we won't prolong her suffering."

The decision to terminate the pregnancy is common in these cases.[6] But there are families who choose to carry to term in spite of an adverse diagnosis. In one study, around 20% of families chose to continue a pregnancy even after receiving a diagnosis of a condition deemed "incompatible with life" (Schectman et al. 2002, 217). Of the families in Benute et al.'s (2012) study, 30.9% chose to continue a pregnancy following a discovery of a lethal fetal malformation (472). Some studies indicate that families who are informed of caregiving options following delivery are more likely to continue the pregnancy. Calhoun et al. (2003) report that 80% of the families in their study chose to continue the pregnancy when informed of comfort care options following birth. D'Almeida et al. (2006) found similar results, noting that 75% of families in their study chose to continue the pregnancy when they were informed of these possibilities.[7] Healthcare providers and medical institutions need to be prepared to support these families.

Perinatal palliative and hospice care is a novel modality of care for families who choose to continue a pregnancy following an adverse diagnosis.[8] In what follows, I use the term 'perinatal hospice' as a stylistic shortening of the more cumbersome 'perinatal palliative and hospice care.' It is important to note, however, that many scholars distinguish between palliative and hospice care. Typically, the term 'palliative' refers to care that ameliorates pain either as a complement to active interventions with targeted curative goals or as a mode of care for patients who have decided to forgo further pursuit of these aims. The term 'hospice' refers to comfort care in contexts where physicians are no longer pursuing curative goals. Hospice care, then, involves the use of palliative measures as an aid to the dying person. For my purposes, I mostly elide this distinction because I focus on cases in which a significantly life-limiting condition renders active interventions unlikely to provide significant therapeutic value. But there are times when this distinction is important because of the prognostic uncertainty attending the diagnosis.[9] In these cases, the planning phase of perinatal hospice involves developing contingency plans for active interventions aimed at sustaining or prolonging life. Thus, my use of the term 'perinatal hospice' should be understood in an expansive sense to cover more than mere comfort care.

Perinatal hospice begins immediately following diagnosis. Physicians provide information to families concerning the care available and the means by which they can secure these measures. The decision to continue a pregnancy initiates a cascade of coordinated activities aimed at preparing for the remainder of the pregnancy, the birth of the child, and post-delivery care. Given the difficulties families face, advanced planning is crucial to facilitating a meaningful experience.

Developing a plan of this kind often involves a team of individuals including obstetricians, neonatologists, nurses, hospital administrators, social workers, counselors, chaplains, and support groups. I typically refer to the team of individuals who act together to extend care as 'healthcare providers.' I employ a general term for stylistic reasons, but the use of this terminology should not be construed as an endorsement of the claim that all of the participants respond to a family in similar ways.[10]

After birth, healthcare providers provide quality medical care fitting to address the child's needs. If death is imminent, the goal is to alleviate pain and suffering while offering a space for families to spend time together. If the child is not actively dying, more aggressive forms of intervention may extend the child's life and reduce suffering. Ideally, physicians engage with the family in shared decision-making, seeking to ensure that the care they offer is both medically appropriate and respectful of the family's values and commitments. Even with significantly life-limiting chromosomal abnormalities like trisomy 18, there are children who defy the odds. For this reason, the medical team and family must adapt their care to the needs of the child—a process that involves attentiveness, flexibility, and clear communication.

Given the likelihood of death or diminished quality of life, however, healthcare providers may be disinclined to consider active measures that could sustain the child's life. The medical team needs to exercise due care in judgments about the futility of treatments and about burdens they may place on the child. After all, debates about the nature of futile and excessively burdensome forms of care are contentious.[11] Individual physicians differ in their judgments about the kinds of care worth pursuing; individual physicians approach end-of-life care in distinct ways. Transparency about the reasons for pursuing active interventions or choosing to forgo these modalities of care is crucial for clear communication and effective shared decision-making.

As a novel extension of end-of-life care, perinatal hospice is a form of fitting care for a child whose prognosis is bleak. It takes both the child and the family into its ambit of concern. It addresses the physical vulnerabilities of a child with a significantly life-limiting condition; it meets parents' needs to care for the child and to be a part of a community that recognizes and values their child. Ideally, it is a form of care that enables the family to experience meaning in the midst of traumatic loss. From the time of diagnosis until the time of natural death, the perinatal hospice team offers supportive care for the entire family. This care extends beyond the child's death to counseling and bereavement care. As a structured program of care, perinatal hospice involves the coordinated and integrated efforts of individuals, groups, and institutions committed to a common project of care.

The aim of this book is to develop a *virtue-based* defense of the value of perinatal hospice.[12] In this chapter, I offer a rationale for this project, highlighting its distinctive commitments and promise. In Section II, I briefly summarize extant analyses of the value of perinatal hospice, noting some important limitations of each of these accounts. My aim is not to refute these analyses; some of the resources my defense provides can be employed to supplement existing defenses. In Section III, I present a sketch of the core commitments of my *virtue-based* defense. In Section IV, I detail a distinctive personal dimension of this work. I am a parent who has benefitted from this form of care. This experience provides important insights into the kinds of goods realized through perinatal hospice. And it grounds an important methodological commitment: each chapter draws on narratives of those who have chosen to continue a pregnancy following an adverse diagnosis. These stories display how perinatal hospice programs meet profound needs through an extension of exemplary care. In Section V, I offer a sketch of the contents of each chapter and conclude by highlighting the distinctive implications one may draw from this *virtue-based* defense of perinatal hospice.

II. On the Value of Perinatal Hospice

There is an expanding body of scholarly literature concerning perinatal hospice, but there have been very few attempts to construct an account of its moral value. Initial discussions of the ethics of perinatal hospice focused on its role as an alternative to abortion. In this context, one can distinguish between two distinct analyses of its value. According to the *moral status* defense, perinatal hospice is valuable because it respects the moral value of the unborn child. The most prominent version of this defense grounds the claim that the unborn child has moral status in a theological account of human dignity. Adopting a specifically Christian perspective, proponents of this account describe the unborn child as a person created in the image of God.[13] Perinatal hospice demonstrates proper respect for the inherent value of human life in its earliest stages by providing an alternative to the violence of abortion.

According to the alternative *reproductive autonomy* defense, the primary good served by perinatal hospice is that it respects the family's choice to continue an affected pregnancy. Proponents of this view maintain that the proper approach to decisions following adverse antenatal diagnosis is to defer to family choices and values. Healthcare providers ought to remain neutral concerning contentious philosophical questions about the nature and value of human life, but they can provide an expanded range of choices aligned with a family's values.

Both of these approaches are limited in important ways.[14] The most prominent species of the *moral status* defense endorses two controversial philosophical views: (i) unborn human life has full moral status and (ii) it has this value because unborn children are created in the image of God. Even if one detaches the account of moral status from theological commitments, the defense is limiting in another way. By focusing exclusively on the moral status of the unborn child, proponents of this account fail to provide a sufficiently expansive framework for understanding the full range of goods realized through perinatal hospice programs.

The *reproductive autonomy* defense is limited in a similar way. Deference to reproductive choices may trigger a suite of practices that honor and validate the family's commitments, but the value of these practices is not fully reducible to respect for reproductive autonomy. Moreover, this defense does not address important questions about whether and the extent to which healthcare providers ought to be deferential to family choices. In some cases, families may desire to prolong life indefinitely without sufficient thought to the potential suffering or burdens this may cause to all of those affected including the healthcare providers. If there are conditions under which deference to family choices is morally problematic, then the value of perinatal hospice cannot be dependent solely upon the value of reproductive autonomy. Finally, proponents of the *reproductive autonomy* defense are committed to the view that the unborn child has no moral status independent of the family's choice to continue the pregnancy. Thus, this view is incompatible with the possibility that the unborn child has inherent moral value.

In addition to these particular limitations, both the *moral status* defense and the *reproductive autonomy* defense are limited by a shared focus on questions at the heart of debates about the ethics of abortion. The value of perinatal hospice is not captured by contrasting it with the alternatives of either abortion or aggressive over-treatment. These accounts focus, at best, on a narrow range of goods manifested in the provision and promotion of perinatal hospice. To underscore this point, consider a parallel discussion. Advocates of hospice care for terminally ill adults may contrast the value of hospice with both physician-assisted suicide and euthanasia and with futile and burdensome interventions, but they do not argue that the primary goods of hospice are reducible to their function as an alternative to these ethically-contested practices. Likewise, proponents of perinatal hospice can and ought to develop accounts of the specific value of perinatal hospice independent of its role as an alternative to the ethically contested practices of either abortion or aggressive over-treatment after birth.

Some scholars and practitioners have offered an account of the moral value of perinatal hospice that goes beyond these analyses—an account that seeks to characterize the wide range of goods realized through this caregiving practice. Although it is perhaps best construed as an extension or development of the *reproductive autonomy* defense, I will call this account the *supportive care* defense.[15] Proponents of this view hold that healthcare providers ought to provide care that adequately addresses the specific needs of patients. If the family chooses to continue the pregnancy, *supportive care* involves planning for the provision of quality end-of-life care for the child after birth. Simultaneously, it involves the extension of *supportive care* to the mother and the family as primary caregivers for the unborn child.

The *supportive care* defense is similar to the *reproductive autonomy* defense in two ways. First, it is predicated on the view that the current range of options for families who receive an adverse diagnosis is unnecessarily restrictive. The options typically presented to the family involve (i) doing nothing, (ii) terminating the pregnancy, or (iii) pursuing aggressive interventions that are potentially futile and often excessively burdensome. For many families, none of these options are tenable. Perinatal hospice is an alternative that avoids the objectionable features of these choices.

Second, it enjoins healthcare providers to adopt a deferential attitude toward the decision to continue or terminate the pregnancy—a decision whose value depends upon the family's conception of the goods realized through this decision. Crucial to this stance is a procedural neutrality expressed in their complete respect for the family's authority in this choice. Clinical neutrality enables healthcare providers to serve families without addressing seemingly intractable philosophical disagreements about the moral status of the unborn child.[16] Feudtner and Munson (2009) observe,

> The ethically appropriate role of the clinician, then, is to acknowledge the prevailing moral indeterminacy of the questions regarding the status of fetuses and appropriate response to their potential future suffering, and to collaborate with the prospective parents in working out well-informed individualized answers to these questions.
>
> (517)

If the family decides to terminate the pregnancy, healthcare providers focus on the mother as the sole patient in their care. Alternatively, the choice to continue the pregnancy acts as a trigger for extending medically appropriate care to both the mother and the unborn child as patients deserving of care. Although this care aligns with the family's choice, it does not imply endorsement of the reasons, values, or commitments (religious or otherwise) grounding parental choice.

In spite of these similarities, the *supportive care* defense differs from the *reproductive autonomy* view because of its recognition of values beyond deference to family choices. Specifically, this view is rooted in a normative conception of quality patient care for the mother, the family, and the unborn child if the family chooses to continue pregnancy. As Steven Leuthner (2004a) notes,

> When the diagnosis of an anomaly is made prenatally, one must keep in mind that there are really two patients for whom decisions must be made. What one decides is appropriate care for an infant after birth likely will affect how one approaches the care of the pregnant woman around the time of delivery.
>
> (748–750)

Importantly, quality medical care does not involve unqualified deference to family choices; there are normative dimensions of apt care grounded in a vision of the proper aims of medicine. In contexts where curative or therapeutic measures cannot benefit the child, healthcare providers seek to ensure comfort and to avoid harm. They weigh decisions about active interventions carefully in order to ensure that they do not subject the child to unnecessary or excessive suffering. Ideally, the goal is to engage with families as genuine partners in shared decision-making. They aim to align fitting care with family values and commitments. When there are conflicting perspectives on the child's best interests, however, healthcare providers must initiate conversations with the family so that they maintain appropriate standards of medical care. Toward this end, the promotion and provision of perinatal hospice can provide crucial support for healthcare providers. As Feudtner and Munson (2009) note, perinatal hospice can help to diminish the possibility of moral distress in circumstances where clinicians feel "compelled to perform invasive procedures on an infant who they perceive as dying" (511).

This account of the value of perinatal hospice improves upon the *reproductive autonomy* defense. It characterizes the value of perinatal hospice in terms of the goods realized in medically appropriate care of patients without reducing its value to a respect for a family's choices. Nonetheless, its neutrality concerning the decision to terminate or continue the pregnancy seems to imply that the unborn child does not have inherent moral status. For proponents of the *supportive care* defense, the unborn child's status as a patient and a fit subject of medical concern is contingent upon the family's decision to continue the pregnancy.[17] But if the unborn child has inherent moral status, its value cannot be predicated upon a family's choice to continue the pregnancy.

Proponents of the *supportive care* defense may respond in at least two ways to this criticism. First, they may accept the view that deference of this sort commits them to the claim that the unborn child lacks inherent moral status but respond that such a commitment is appropriate because of other clinical goals. Crucially, it prevents a clinician from pressuring families to comply with his preferred choice options. Thus, the clinician does not undercut the family's proper legal authority over a private decision. Second, they may reject the claim that deference to the family's choice commits them to the view that the unborn child lacks inherent moral worth. Instead, it commits them to the view that the best way to honor the value of the unborn child as a patient is to defer to the family's decision concerning what is in the child's best interest. Decisions about the child's best interests are not under the sole discretion of clinicians; it requires conversations with the child's primary caregivers. If families and physicians together determine that it would be in the best interest of the unborn child to terminate the pregnancy, it is not clear that this violates the respect due to the unborn child as a patient with moral worth.

Both of these responses commit supporters of the *supportive care* defense to contested claims. The first response acknowledges a commitment to a contested philosophical position about moral status but maintains that this stance is appropriate because of the family's legal authority over private decisions. As a matter of law, this response may be adequate. But as a response to moral questions concerning the practice of medicine, it is not sufficient. The second response is better in addressing moral questions, but it involves endorsing the view that the ongoing life of the unborn child is worse for the child than its immediate death. Although there are some contexts where this may seem true, proponents of this view need to offer additional argument in support of the claim that death can be in the best interests of a child.

Proponents of the extant analyses I have outlined in this section may be able to develop their respective views in ways that address the limitations I have noted. But the limitations I have discussed suggest that contemporary accounts of the value of perinatal hospice need supplemental development and defense. My goal in this work is not to refute or supplant these approaches; in fact, the account I articulate in this book may provide resources to supplement or extend these approaches. To the extent that there are aspects of my defense that are compatible with alternative analyses, proponents of other views can draw on my discussion to deepen their own accounts. In the final chapter, I return to this comparative analysis, offering an extended discussion of the merits of the *virtue-based* defense relative to the extant analyses.

In what follows, I develop an alternative vision of the value of this novel form of care—an account that seeks to characterize the full range of goods realized through this novel form of care. My defense is an extended work of applied virtue ethics. It seeks to shed light on the ways individual healthcare providers, professional communities, and institutions realize important moral goods through a collective effort to care for affected families. Individuals and institutions who join together in this way contribute to an ethos of exemplary care.

III. Central Commitments of This Defense

The central claim I seek to defend in this work is the following: perinatal hospice is a common project of care that manifests virtues essential to addressing substantive human needs.[18] Virtues are human excellences, the possession and exercise of which are crucial for human fulfillment.[19] At the individual level, virtues are stable, enduring, and deeply entrenched traits that dispose a person to feel, to act, and to reason well in a wide range of trait-relevant circumstances. In this section, I outline three of the key commitments of this project, postponing a full development until the next chapter.

The first commitment of this work is a commitment to the view that some virtues are particularly attuned to human vulnerability—that is, they take human need as a focal object of concern. This is the central insight I draw from Alasdair MacIntyre's (1999a) account of the virtues of acknowledged dependence. These virtues are habits of concerned attention to and vigilant care for human vulnerability. A person who possesses these virtues is disposed to recognize his indebtedness to the care of others and to commit himself to caring for the needs of others. These virtues shape communities in ways that help them to realize genuine human goods. Perhaps most importantly, the possession and exercise of these virtues enables communities to promote and provide for those whose needs are greatest.[20] There are a number of implications one may draw from this account, but one point deserves emphasis: the activities, behaviors, and thoughts of individuals and communities who fail to possess and exercise these virtues disproportionately affect those who are most vulnerable. These failures add to the difficulties experienced by those whose vulnerabilities are extensive and profound.

I contend that perinatal hospice manifests virtues crucial for identifying, recognizing, appreciating, and addressing the vulnerabilities and needs occasioned by a significantly life-limiting *in utero* diagnosis. I focus on four virtues: hospitality, hope, solidarity, and compassion. Each of these dispositions take particular human needs as a central object of concern. The need for welcome is a focal concern of the virtue of hospitality. The need for meaningful possibilities worthy of pursuit is a focal concern of the virtue of hope. The need for human presence is a focal concern of the virtue of solidarity. The need for consolation in grief is a focal concern of the virtue of compassion. In the central chapters of this work, I provide extended profiles of each of these virtues in the previously articulated order. The central reason why I adopt this order is that it draws attention to salient features of a family's needs as they emerge in the time between diagnosis and death. The need for both welcome and meaning is often salient immediately following the diagnosis. The need for accompaniment becomes salient as families seek to navigate social and institutional spaces as they wait. The need for consolation takes on special significance in the finality of death.

Two clarificatory remarks are necessary in this context. First, throughout this work, I consider the needs of parents or families considered primarily *as a unit*. I do not deny that there are important differences in the distinct needs of particular family members. Even when there are common needs, the ways mothers, fathers, siblings, and extended family experience these needs may vary considerably. Thus, it is important to note potential differences between the needs of mothers and fathers, between the needs of single mothers and parents who are married, between parents and siblings of the affected child, and between parents and the extended family. Appreciating these differences can enable individuals and professional communities to care for each individual and the specific vulnerabilities he or she experiences.

Second, although I focus on the distinct virtues within each of the central chapters, there are a number of practices that simultaneously exhibit multiple virtues. One explanation of this phenomenon is that some virtues cluster together because of their allied functions in a person's character. Here, I endorse Gulliford and Roberts's (2018) claim that there are *virtues of intelligent caring* grounded in a motivated concern for important moral goods—that is, the substantive concerns of morality.[21] Among these virtues are dispositions that are grounded in a benevolent concern for another's wellbeing. Compassion and gratitude, for instance, each involve an allocentric orientation of benevolence toward another person.[22] Although each are distinct, they are integrated in important ways within a virtuous person's life in orienting him to the pursuit of the good or wellbeing of others.

Three of these virtues I describe in my *virtue-based* defense of perinatal hospice are natural members of this allocentric cluster. Hospitality, solidarity, and compassion are each rooted in an intelligent and caring concern for the wellbeing of others. The fourth virtue, hope, is better construed as an *emotion-virtue*—that is, a virtue for well-tuned emotional appraisal concerning desired outcomes that are good but difficult to secure. Some expressions of this virtue, however, can draw upon an abiding concern for the wellbeing of others. One expression of virtuous hope is an allocentric hope on another's behalf. I contend that hospitality, allocentric hope, solidarity, and compassion cluster together in important ways. A corollary of this claim is that failures to express one of these virtues are often failures in the expression of closely aligned traits. In this book, I argue that this specific allocentric cluster is crucial to addressing the needs of families affected by an adverse *in utero* diagnosis.

Even if these virtues are united by a common allocentric concern, each chapter of the book offers an account of the distinct ways these individual virtues are crucial to meeting specific needs. So, it is important to show how one can individuate these distinct expressions of allocentric concern. Although I must bracket extended discussion until later chapters, it is important to forecast some of the later developments here.

For the purpose of this work, I note two primary ways one can distinguish between individual members of this cluster of virtues: (i) they are each responsive to distinct kinds of need and (ii) they each issue in distinctive patterns of thought, feeling, and activity. Consider first how these virtues are responsive to distinct needs. Hospitality is a virtue of caring concern for a person who is vulnerable because of *his social exclusion and a lack of standing within a community*. Allocentric hope is a virtue of caring concern for a person who is vulnerable because of his *susceptibility to hopelessness or despair in conditions where there are available goods worthy of continued pursuit*. Solidarity is a virtue of caring concern for a person who is vulnerable because of *his isolation in the midst of hardship*. Compassion is a virtue of caring concern for a person who is vulnerable *because of his serious suffering*. In short, each of these virtues is responsive to a particular kind of human vulnerability.

The fact that these virtues are responsive to distinct types of needs has important implications for the factors that are salient or striking in the virtuous person's construal of the situation. These sensitivities reflect one's attunement to distinct types of eliciting condition. Hospitality primes one to see those who are excluded and on the margins; allocentric hope attunes one to see those who are in danger of despair; solidarity makes one sensitive to those who are alone and longing for companionship; compassion trains one vision toward those who are suffering and in need of comfort. If a person's estrangement or social exclusion is salient, it will elicit hospitality—a concern to invite and welcome the other in to a space of belonging and care. If a person's nearing hopelessness or despair is salient, it will elicit allocentric hope—a hope extended as a support to the other for the maintenance and exercise of fitting hope in conditions of anticipated disappointment. If a person's isolation or solitude is salient, it will elicit solidarity—a concern to be with the other in solidarity. If a person's suffering is salient, this will elicit compassion—a concern to take on the project of co-suffering with the individual in need.

A second way one can distinguish between the distinct members of this allocentric cluster is by focusing on their characteristic expressions. Hospitality moves the person to invite and welcome the stranger into a space of belonging and protection as a guest. Allocentric hope moves the person to hold out a vision of potential goods and the routes to their realization as a supportive scaffolding for the maintenance or recovery of another's hope. Solidarity moves the person to address a person's isolation by moving toward the person to be with him so that he is not alone. Compassion moves the person to take up the suffering of another individual as his own.

Although one can distinguish the virtues in these ways, there are important interdependencies and connections between these traits. Given the common basis in a concern for the wellbeing of others, acts that express one of these virtues (e.g., hospitality) can simultaneously express allocentric hope (e.g., in facilitating hope for those whose social exclusion make them susceptible to hopelessness and despair), solidarity (e.g., in addressing the isolation commonly co-occurring with social alienation and feelings of hopelessness), and compassion (e.g., in addressing the suffering resulting from social exclusion, hopelessness, and isolation). Likewise, the failure to express one of these virtues (e.g., compassion) can be a simultaneous failure to express hospitality (e.g., in failing to display a proper sensitivity to the serious suffering that results from social exclusion), allocentric hope (e.g., in failing to provide support for the hope that there are goods worth pursuing even in the midst of suffering), and solidarity (e.g., in failing to display a willingness to be with the person who is suffering because of his isolation). Given that varied forms of vulnerability are commonly co-occurring, the virtuous person's construal of the individual in need will be a complex construal of one who is simultaneously *alienated*, *isolated*, *suffering*, and *potentially without hope*. Thus, virtues move persons and communities to address each of the aspects of the complex experience of need.

A second commitment of my defense is that adequately responding to substantive moral tasks often requires the collaborative efforts of individuals, communities, and institutions. The needs of families in contexts of life-limiting *in utero* diagnoses are a paradigmatic instance of this kind. Physicians may have vital competencies to address particular medical concerns in establishing a plan of adequate care after birth, but it is too much to expect them to attend to the full range of the family's needs. Physicians need the support of other caregivers to help care for the psychosocial needs families experience following diagnosis. Furthermore, individual caregivers need institutional support to promote and provide this kind of care when external social factors create barriers to ensuring care. Properly addressing the needs of the family thus involves individual, communal, and institutional participation in a collaborative project. Or, to put it slightly differently, it involves a shared commitment to a good common project.

In this context, I draw upon Robert Adams's (2006) account of common projects. Adams argues that one of the most basic features of human sociality is engagement in projects "we share with other people" (Adams 2006, 85). From our work with colleagues to our collaborative efforts as parents to our participation on teams or partnerships, many of the most important forms of social interaction are embedded within common projects. Given the centrality of common projects, Adams contends that "caring, in an appropriate way, about good common projects for their own sake is morally virtuous" (2006, 86). It is a virtue both because it is a way of *being for* good projects and because it is a way of *being for* others—a kind of allocentric orientation that is expressive of a central good of human life.[23] I maintain that it is fitting to ascribe virtues to the professional communities that promote and provide perinatal hospice in virtue of their caring commitment to this good common project.[24]

A third commitment of my defense is that one may ascribe excellences to the social structures of an institution. One can think of social structures as "durable systems of patterned social interaction" that frame and constrain interactions between and among individuals (Smith 2010, 322).[25] Some social structures are internal to the institutions of medical care—defined roles, protocols, and policies that delineate how actors within the institutions achieve the goals of an institution. Furthermore, some of these structures are rooted in the physical environment in which families and physicians interact (e.g., the medical examination room). These material spaces encode and embed particular kinds of social engagement actors construe as fitting for the circumstances. There are also social structures external to institutions (e.g., legal norms or broadly shared cultural attitudes) that either frame or interact with institutional structures in ways that can impact interactions between patients and healthcare providers.

Generally, we might call social structures virtuous if they facilitate or encourage individual and communal participation in care that manifests virtues responsive to human vulnerability.[26] Conversely, one can argue that some communities or institutions fail to hit the mark in responding to the needs of affected families. Social structures within communities and institutions may fail to manifest virtue or may actively promote vice. These failures can hinder a family's ability to cope with a devastating diagnosis. Focusing on these kinds of institutional and structural deficiencies provides a clear mode of diagnosing contemporary social structures and practices that add to the burdens of affected families. Experiences within medical settings following the diagnosis of a significantly life-limiting condition can be exceptionally difficult, adding suffering to an already traumatic loss. But it is important to note that these kinds of deficient care are not always a result of vice displayed by individual healthcare providers. Individuals within these institutions may be reliably discharging their role in accordance with social structures that are deficient.

IV. The Personal Is the Philosophical[27]

Before outlining the content of each of the remaining chapters, it is important to highlight one additional feature that makes this book distinctive within the available literature on perinatal hospice. My perspective on these issues is informed by the experience of benefitting from this form of care. My son, Samuel, was born on January 1, 2012 and died in the early morning hours of January 2, 2012. He lived the entirety of his short nearly five-hour life in the back corner of a neonatal intensive care unit (NICU), cloistered in the loving care of his family and friends. He had trisomy 18 and a constellation of other physical limitations: a severe omphalocele, underdeveloped lungs, holes in his heart, and significantly diminished growth (at birth, he weighed just under four pounds).[28] My wife carried Samuel for a little over three months after receiving his official diagnosis; for just over 100 days, we prepared simultaneously for his birth and his death.

The fetal-maternal specialist who diagnosed Samuel suggested that we could 'interrupt' the pregnancy; but, otherwise, she told us there was nothing they could do for us.[29] Terminating the pregnancy was not a live option for our family. So, we turned to my wife's obstetrician to help craft a plan of care. She helped us to develop a plan that honored our time with Sam. When the time came for his delivery, the care we received at the hospital was unwaveringly supportive. Our obstetrician had already briefed the neonatologist, the nurses in labor and delivery, and the caregivers in the NICU about the care we desired. I was able to sit briefly with the neonatologist and communicate the plan we had developed, discussing the commitments crucial to our requests. We wanted nonaggressive care including oxygen support with nasal cannula and pain medication to address any potential discomfort. If possible, we wanted the opportunity to introduce Samuel to family and friends. And we wanted the opportunity to recalibrate these plans if the conditions warranted more active forms of intervention.

The physicians and the nurses involved in our care honored all of these requests. This professional community worked tirelessly through the night to provide care for Samuel and for our whole family. The care we received both immediately after his birth and throughout his short life was seamless. We were able to introduce him to friends; we were able to participate in important religious rites. In his final moments, everyone in the NICU from the healthcare providers to our family and friends were present with us. It was a profoundly sad experience, but it was also an experience of profound love, peace, and meaning. And memories of this experience, the care we received, and our final moments with Sam are overwhelmingly and unequivocally good.[30]

My perspective as a father and spouse informs arguments throughout the book. This perspective has made me sensitive to both the shared experience of vulnerability and the distinct ways members of a family may experience common needs. Although my wife Alisha and I experienced common concerns, addressing her needs required attending to the physical, emotional, and social demands of a difficult pregnancy. I have no doubt that her experience of the need for welcome, meaning, accompaniment, and consolation differed from my own. Furthermore, our needs as parents differed from the needs of our son Micah who was four years old at the time Sam was diagnosed. This has become more salient to me in the years following Sam's death as Micah wrestles with his personal grief over the loss of his brother.

The situated quality of my understanding of the value of perinatal hospice, however, invites a potential objection concerning the personal qualities of this book. Many philosophers maintain that one ought to approach contested questions in ethics from an impersonal, or neutral, stance—that is, the proper approach to disputed questions requires detachment from emotional or intimate investment with the subjects under dispute. This normative stance enables one to consider and to weigh evidence and arguments free from the potentially biasing effects of personal attachments and experience.

Although this is an important concern, there are reasons to challenge the assumption implicit in this meta-philosophical stance. Consider two recent criticisms of this stance from literature on the philosophy of disability. As a philosopher with a physical disability, Elizabeth Barnes (2016) describes an initial hesitancy to write about disability because of the personal nature of the work. She writes,

> But on reflection, that's absurd. Disability is a topic that's personal for everyone. The last time I checked, most non-disabled people are pretty personally invested in being non-disabled. The fact that this sort of personal investment is so easy to ignore is one of the more pernicious aspects of philosophy's obsession with objective neutrality. It's easy to confuse the view from normal with the view from nowhere. And then it's uniquely the minority voices which we single out as biased or lacking objectivity. When it comes to disability, I'm not objective. And neither are you. And that's true whether you're disabled or (temporarily) non-disabled.
>
> (ix)

Thus, Barnes contends that the pursuit of 'objective neutrality' is bound to fail.

Similarly, Eva Kittay (2009) contends that attachments to individuals with profound cognitive impairments (such as her own daughter, Sesha) can give one privileged epistemic access to truths about personhood. She writes, "The close attentive eye needed to care for the dependent individual gives rise to perceptual capabilities that are not shared by those who have at best a glancing acquaintance" (620). The supposed 'objectivity' of a detached perspective may prevent one from seeing or appreciating the relevant values at stake. Taken together, these criticisms provide reasons to interrogate the implicit meta-philosophical commitment to detachment as the appropriate stance from which to philosophize about important and contested issues in applied ethics. Detachment has important virtues, but it can limit one's perspective by restricting the range of potential evidence.

Nonetheless, I am sensitive to the concern that my experiences are potentially epistemically biasing. Proximity of this sort may skew my perspective, leading me to adopt conclusions I am antecedently inclined to endorse. So, in what follows, I seek to address this concern in two ways. First, my argument draws on a range of evidence beyond my own experience. In particular, it engages with the expanding literature on the experiences of families who continue pregnancies following an adverse diagnosis. Second, I attend to narratives of families other than my own, noting the ways their stories illuminate a common set of concerns. I give voice to the experiences of these families because there is something to be learned from attending carefully to those who have been most affected by significantly life-limiting diagnoses.

V. Conclusion—An Outline of the Book

This work is the first philosophical monograph exclusively focused on perinatal hospice. But the implications of the framework I develop are broader than this targeted inquiry may suggest. The work as a whole advances scholarly discussion in several ways. First, it displays the value of applied virtue ethics as a constructive form of ethical inquiry. For a significant period of time, the subdisciplines of applied and practical ethics have been dominated by consequentialist and deontological frameworks. As Nancy Snow (2018) observes, "The emergence of virtue ethics adds exciting new dimensions to [practical and applied ethics]" (4). My defense offers a portrait of this novel and exciting approach to applied ethics.

Second, this work draws upon important but underexplored resources for applied ethics. For instance, MacIntyre's account of the virtues of acknowledged dependence has been influential in philosophical discussions of virtues, but it has not been brought to bear on the particular issues addressed in this book. My defense provides an important resource for thinking about the relationship between need, vulnerability, and the tasks expressive of virtue. Additionally, reflection on virtuous common projects provides a fruitful way of thinking about virtue writ large within social groups, organizations, institutions, and social structures. These discussions can advance our thinking about projects of structural and institutional reform as crucial exercises of virtuous concern.

Third, the framework I develop in this work may have consequences for debates and questions beyond those I discuss in these pages. Thinking carefully about the virtues of hospitality, hope, solidarity, and compassion could help to frame our thinking about end-of-life care in general. For instance, debates about physician-assisted suicide and euthanasia often draw upon the language of compassion, but more attention ought to be devoted to the distinct conceptions of compassion that underpin these contentious disputes.[31] Additionally, reflections on these virtues may have implications for debates about the ethical use of prenatal screening, disability selective abortion and eugenics, and questions about the normative relationship between parents and their children.

Furthermore, there may be implications for debates beyond the domain of biomedical ethics. Serious reflection upon the virtues of hospitality, solidarity, and compassion may contribute to applied ethics discussions about, for instance, the proper forms of care and concern for individuals with disability or for refugees and immigrants. Thus, this work of applied virtue ethics has potential to deepen reflection upon moral questions of significant contemporary concern.

Finally, and perhaps most importantly, the arguments of this work could help both practitioners and advocates of perinatal hospice to understand its value more clearly. A grasp of the goods this form of care makes possible can enable practitioners to extend their caregiving in ways that meet profound needs. It can provide a rationale for the pursuit of crucial reforms within medical institutions and beyond. In this way, the arguments of this work can help to contribute to a culture that better meets the profound needs of families facing an adverse *in utero* diagnosis.

The central chapters of this book are dedicated to developing and defending the claim that perinatal hospice is a good common project of care that manifests virtues that can address the needs of those facing a significantly life-limiting diagnosis. The structure of the book as a whole is as follows. In Chapter 2, I begin by providing an extended account of the central philosophical and methodological commitments enumerated briefly in this chapter. I frame my discussion of the relations between virtue and human vulnerability by offering a sketch of MacIntyre's account of the virtues of acknowledged dependence. Then, I detail Robert Adams's analysis of virtuous common projects. Finally, I offer a discussion of the grounds for ascribing virtues or their corresponding vices to both institutions and social structures.

In Chapter 3, I focus on the initial diagnosis of a significantly life-limiting condition, the need for welcome it engenders, and the ways perinatal hospice can address this need. The central aim of this chapter is to show how perinatal hospice manifests the virtue of hospitality. I offer a map of the virtue of hospitality, contrasting it with a range of associated vices including hostility and indifference. I also distinguish between genuine hospitality and several counterfeit expressions of hospitable welcome. Finally, I contrast the hospitable ethos of perinatal hospice programs with the inhospitable culture many families face following diagnosis. I conclude with a brief discussion of the ways one might cultivate a more hospitable institutional culture.

In Chapter 4, I note how a diagnosis of a significantly life-limiting condition creates a need for meaning in the face of almost certain disappointment and sorrow. The central aim of this chapter is to argue that perinatal hospice scaffolds a family's hope in the pursuit of meaningful possibilities. I contend that the provision of this supportive structure for a family's hope is itself an expression of the virtue of hope, a trait I contrast with several related anticipatory emotions and the vices of presumption and despair. Furthermore, I consider evidence of the ways in which common institutional practices can fail to sustain a family's capacity for well-tuned hope or, worse, facilitate a sense of hopelessness. I conclude this chapter with a brief discussion of how one might cultivate an institutional culture that promotes hope in families struggling to find meaning in the midst of anticipated loss.

In Chapter 5, I attend to the family's need for individuals and institutions that accompany them as they endure the time between diagnosis and death. Families often report feeling isolated and abandoned in their need; solitude can make the experience of continuing a pregnancy particularly challenging. In order to address this vulnerability, they need to know that they are not alone. I seek to show how perinatal hospice expresses the virtue of solidarity, a virtue of kind and attentive accompaniment. I contrast this virtue with several species of vice, all of which move a person to resist or detach from a union characteristic of solidary bonds. I maintain that perinatal hospice programs establish an ethos in which families experience genuine solidarity. And I contrast this with a climate of abandonment and isolation affecting those families who receive adverse *in utero* diagnoses. I conclude this chapter with a brief discussion of how one might cultivate an institutional culture that promotes solidarity with families facing an adverse diagnosis.

In Chapter 6, I focus on the family's need for bereavement care. Much of the experience following an adverse diagnosis could be construed as a process of coming to terms with the myriad losses a family experiences. They grieve the loss of (i) a normal pregnancy, (ii) their status or identity as a family, (iii) attachments and bonds, (iv) caregiving opportunities, (v) the ability to fulfill vital roles as a parent (e.g., protecting, nurturing, and soothing the child), (vi) future dreams, goals, wishes, hopes, and expectations for the child, (vii) the child's life after death, and (viii) the support of caregivers after they leave the hospital. In order to address these needs, individuals and institutions ought to exercise the virtue of compassion, a disposition that manifests itself in the consoling work of suffering with and for others. I contrast this virtue with the vices of excessive or deficient concern for the suffering of others. The chapter shows how perinatal hospice programs enact compassionate consolation for those who grieve, contrasting this kind of exemplary care with current institutional structures that fail to address the bereavement needs of families. The chapter closes with a discussion of the ways one may foster institutional support for the development and expression of these compassionate forms of consolation.

In Chapter 7, I summarize the central argument of the book, highlighting the distinctive dimensions of my *virtue-based* defense of perinatal hospice. One of the important implications of my argument is that a concern for virtue provides a rationale for healthcare providers, professional communities, and institutions to promote and provide perinatal hospice. But there are structures and attitudes that can inhibit this kind of work. In this chapter, I identify and seek to address some of the obstacles that hinder reforms crucial to promoting and providing care.

I consider barriers arising from an insufficient understanding of perinatal hospice to the lack of funding to the politicization of care to attitudinal commitments concerning the burdens of suffering and disability. I argue that common projects of social and institutional reform to remove these obstacles can be a substantive response to the summons of virtue to promote exemplary care.

Notes

1 Norwitz and Levy (2013) note that new noninvasive testing promises to find a host of markers for disability as early as ten weeks into a pregnancy.
2 There are scholarly debates concerning whether such a choice expresses a devaluation of the lives of those living with disabilities. For discussion, see Parens and Asch (2000); Reinders (2000); and Wasserman, Wachbroit, and Bickenbach (2005).
3 Trisomy 18 occurs in roughly 1 out of 2,500 of pregnancies, but only approximately 1 in 8,000 of affected pregnancies result in a live birth. For individuals with full trisomy 18, each cell of the body has an extra copy of the eighteenth chromosome. Some individuals have mosaic, or partial, trisomy 18. For these individuals, some cells have the usual two copies of the eighteenth chromosome while others have a third copy.
4 See www.trisomy18.org/what-is-trisomy-18/ for more details.
5 For recent discussion concerning active interventions after birth and their import for improving life-expectancy for children born with trisomy 18, see Andrews et al. (2016); Bruns (2013); Janvier and Watkins (2013); Janvier, Farlow, and Barrington (2016); Kosho et al. (2013); McCaffrey (2016); and Meyer et al. (2016).
6 For evidence that the majority of families choose to terminate pregnancies following diagnoses of these kinds, see Benute et al. (2012); Hassed et al. (1993); Lakovschek, Streubel, and Ulm (2011); Sandelowski and Barroso (2005); Sandelowski and Jones (1996); Schectman et al. (2002); Wilkinson et al. (2012); and Wool (2011).
7 Two other studies Breeze et al. (2007) and Leuthner and Jones (2007) report higher percentages (40% and 37% respectively) than one would expect from earlier studies. For some critical discussion of these studies see, Balaguer et al. (2012).
8 Although there are numerous perinatal hospice programs throughout the United States (and in more than twenty countries around the world), awareness of and access to these forms of care is limited. For a list of available programs, see www.perinatalhospice.org. For discussion of the development of perinatal hospice, see Balaguer et al. (2012); Bhatia (2006); Calhoun and Hoeldtke (1996); Calhoun et al. (2003); Calhoun, Reitman, and Hoeldtke (1997); Carter and Bhatia (2001); Catlin and Carter (2002); Chitty, Barnes, and Berry (1996); Cobb (2016); Collier (2011); D'Almeida et al. (2006); Hoeldtke and Calhoun (2001); Kuebelbeck and Davis (2011); Leuthner (2004a, 2004b); Leuthner and Jones (2007); Munson and Leuthner (2007); Ramer-Chrastek and Thygeson (2005); Roush et al. (2007); Sumner, Kavanaugh, and Moro (2006); Whitfield, Siegel, and Glicken (1982); Williams et al. (2008); and Wool (2011, 2013a).
9 This is most relevant in Chapter 4.
10 There may be important differences in how individuals acting within various roles react to affected families. At specific points in this work, I note relevant and available evidence concerning these differences.

11 There are significant disagreements about how one ought to understand 'futile' treatments. For discussions, see Aghabarary and Nayeri (2016); Brody and Halevy (1995); Helft, Siegler, and Lantos (2000); Schneiderman, Jecker, and Jonsen (1990); Wilkinson and Savulescu (2011); and Wilkinson et al. (2012).

12 In Chapter 2, I explicitly distinguish between the formal structures and practices characteristic of perinatal hospice and virtuous perinatal hospice programs. But throughout the book as a whole, I often employ the term 'perinatal hospice' as a success term—that is, as a shorthand for virtuous perinatal hospice programs.

13 See Calhoun and Hoeldtke (1996) for a clear statement of this defense. Calhoun, Reitman, and Hoeldtke (1997) offer a related defense.

14 This is a development of criticisms I initially advanced in Cobb (2016).

15 For a clear expression of this type of account, see, Feudtner and Munson (2009). For analyses emphasizing similar principles, see Marty and Carter (2018) and Wool (2013b).

16 For further discussion, see Yoon, Rasinski, and Curlin (2010).

17 For criticism, see Watt (2017).

18 My account differs in important ways from Williams's (2015) virtue-based defense. I describe these differences in Chapter 2.

19 Although I endorse a *eudaimonistic* account of the nature of the virtues, the core of my argument is independent of this commitment. At a minimum, what is required for my defense is that the virtues to which I point are forms of human excellence expressive of moral and personal goodness.

20 MacIntyre's (1999a) work focuses primarily upon the needs of those with profound disabilities. For critical engagement with MacIntyre, see Poore (2014).

21 One can distinguish these *virtues of intelligent caring* from what Roberts (1989) calls *virtues of willpower, virtues of detachment*, and *emotion-virtues*. *Virtues of willpower*, or *structural virtues*, are dispositions that enable one to address those emotions or concerns that frustrate or inhibit one's pursuit of moral goods. The *virtues of detachment* are dispositions for an absence of a range of affective responses. Humility, for instance, is a virtue of detachment that frees one from an excessive concern for self-elevation or self-importance. *Emotion-virtues* are dispositions for the expression of characteristically appropriate emotions within a particular situation.

22 Other virtues, like humility, are necessary for the expression of allocentric virtues because a concern for self-importance can prevent one from caring properly for others.

23 Adams (2006) defines virtue as an excellence in *being for* the good. In what follows, I assume that a *eudaimonistic* account of the virtues can accommodate much of what Adams says about common projects.

24 There is a growing body of literature concerning collective virtues that supports such ascriptions. See, for instance, Beggs (2003); Byerly and Byerly (2016); Fricker (2010); Lahroodi (2007); MacIntyre (1999b); Sandin (2007); Smith (1982); and Ziv (2012). For recent criticism of the notion of group virtues, see Cordell (2016).

25 For an analysis of distinct account of social structures, see Porpora (1989).

26 See Anderson (2012) and Fricker (2010) for additional discussion.

27 This heading is a specific reference to Kittay (2009).

28 An omphalocele is an abdominal wall defect in which the internal organs are encased within a sac outside of abdominal wall. In Sam's case, the size of the omphalocele significantly compromised his lung function.

29 It is important to note the euphemistic nature of the term 'interrupt.' Multiple physicians used this language in the description of our options.
30 See Cobb (2014) for further discussion of our experience.
31 See S. Kay Toombs (2018) for a helpful discussion of divergent views of compassion for these debates.

References

Adams, Robert. 2006. *A Theory of Virtue: Excellence in Being for the Good.* Oxford: Clarendon Press.

Aghabarary, Maryam and Hahid Dehghan Nayeri. 2016. "Medical Futility and Its Challenges: A Review Study." *Journal of Medical Ethics and History of Medicine* 9 (11): 1–13.

Anderson, Elizabeth. 2012. "Epistemic Justice as a Virtue of Social Institutions." *Social Epistemology* 26 (2): 163–73.

Andrews, Sasha E., Ann G. Downey, David Scott Showalter, Heather Fitzgerald, Vivian P. Showalter, John C. Carey, and Peter Hulac. 2016. "Shared Decision Making and the Pathways Approach in the Prenatal and Postnatal Management of the Trisomy 13 and Trisomy 18 Syndromes." *American Journal of Medical Genetics Part C: Seminars in Medical Genetics* 172 (3): 257–63.

Balaguer, Albert, Ana Martín-Ancel, Darío Ortigoza-Escobar, Joaquín Escribano, and Josep Argemi. 2012. "The Model of Palliative Care in the Perinatal Setting: A Review of the Literature." *BMC Pediatrics* 12 (1): 1–7.

Barnes, Elizabeth. 2016. *The Minority Body: A Theory of Disability.* New York: Oxford University Press.

Beggs, Donald. 2003. "The Idea of Group Moral Virtue." *Journal of Social Philosophy* 34 (3): 457–74.

Benute, Gláucia R.G., Roseli M.Y. Nomura, Adolfo W. Liao, Maria de Lourdes Brizot, Mara de Lucia, and M. Zugaib. 2012. "Feelings of Women Regarding End-of-life Decision Making after Ultrasound Diagnosis of a Lethal Fetal Malformation." *Midwifery* 28 (4): 472–5.

Bhatia, J. 2006. "Palliative Care in the Fetus and Newborn." *Journal of Perinatology* 26 (S1): S24–S26.

Breeze, Andrew C.G., Christopher C. Lees, Arvind Kumar, Hannah H. Missfelder-Lobos, and Edile M. Murdoch. 2007. "Palliative Care for Prenatally Diagnosed Lethal Fetal Abnormality." *Archives of Disease in Childhood-Fetal and Neonatal Edition* 92 (1): F56–F58.

Brody, Baruch A. and Amir Halevy. 1995. "Is Futility a Futile Concept?" *The Journal of Medicine and Philosophy* 20 (2): 123–44.

Bruns, Deborah J. 2013. "Erring on the Side of Life: Children with Rare Trisomy Conditions, Medical Interventions and the Quality of Life." *Journal of Genetic Disorders & Genetic Reports* 2 (1): 1–4.

Byerly, T. Ryan and Meghan Byerly. 2016. "Collective Virtue." *The Journal of Value Inquiry* 50 (1): 33–50.

Calhoun, Byron C. and Nathan J. Hoeldtke. 1996. "The Perinatal Hospice." *Journal of Biblical Ethics in Medicine* 9 (1): 20–3.

Calhoun, Byron C., James S. Reitman, and Nathan J. Hoeldtke. 1997. "Perinatal Hospice: A Response to Partial Birth Abortion for Infants with Congenital Defects." *Issues in Law & Medicine* 13: 125–43.

Calhoun, Byron C., Peter Napolitano, Melisa Terry, Carie Bussy, and Nathan J. Hoeldke. 2003. "Perinatal Hospice: Comprehensive Care for the Family of the Fetus with a Lethal Condition." *Obstetrical & Gynecological Survey* 58 (11): 718–19.

Carter, Brian S. and Jatinder Bhatia. 2001. "Comfort/Palliative Care Guidelines for Neonatal practice: Development and Implementation in an Academic Medical Center." *Journal of Perinatology* 21 (5): 279–83.

Catlin, Anita and Brian Carter. 2002. "Creation of a Neonatal End-of-life Palliative Care Protocol." *Neonatal Network: The Journal of Neonatal Nursing* 22 (3): 37–49.

Chitty, Lyn S., Chris A. Barnes, and Caroline Berry. 1996. "Continuing with Pregnancy After a Diagnosis of Lethal Abnormality: Experience of Five Couples and Recommendations for Management." *BMJ: British Medical Journal* 313 (7055): 478–80.

Cobb, Aaron D. 2014. *Loving Samuel: Suffering, Dependence, and the Calling of Love*. Eugene: Cascade Books.

Cobb, Aaron D. 2016. "Acknowledged Dependence and the Virtues of Perinatal Hospice." *Journal of Medicine and Philosophy* 41 (1): 25–40.

Collier, Roger. 2011. "Providing Hospice in the Womb." *Canadian Medical Association Journal* 183: E267–E268.

Cordell, Sean. 2016. "Group Virtues: No Great Leap Forward with Collectivism." *Res Publica* 23 (1): 43–59.

D'Almeida, Michelle, R.F. Hume, Anthony Lathrop, Adaku Njoku, and Byron C. Calhoun. 2006. "Perinatal Hospice: Family-centered Care of the Fetus with a Lethal Condition." *Journal of American Physicians and Surgeons* 11 (2): 52–5.

Feudtner, Chris and David Munson. 2009. "The Ethics of Perinatal Palliative Care." In *The Penn Center Guide to Bioethics*, edited by A. Fiester, and A.L. Caplan, 509–18. New York: Springer.

Fricker, Miranda. 2010. "Can There Be Institutional Virtues?" In *Oxford Studies in Epistemology, Social Epistemology*, edited by Tamar Szabo Gendler and John Hawthorne, 235–52. Oxford: Oxford University Press.

Gulliford, Liz and Robert C. Roberts. 2018. "Exploring the 'Unity' of the Virtues: The Case of an Allocentric Quintet." *Theory & Psychology* 28 (2): 208–26.

Hassed, Susan J., Connie H. Miller, Sandra K. Pope, Pamela Murphy, J. Gerald Quirk, Jr., and Christopher Cunniff. 1993. "Perinatal Lethal Conditions: The Effect of Diagnosis on Decision Making." *Obstetrics & Gynecology* 82 (1): 37–42.

Helft, Paul R., Mark Siegler, and John Lantos. 2000. "The Rise and Fall of the Futility Movement." *The New England Journal of Medicine* 343: 206–93.

Hoeldtke, Nathan J. and Byron C. Calhoun. 2001. "Perinatal Hospice." *American Journal of Obstetrics and Gynecology* 185 (3): 525–9.

Janvier, Annie and Andrew Watkins. 2013. "Medical Interventions for Children with Trisomy 13 and Trisomy 18: What is the Value of a Short Disabled Life?" *Acta Paediatrica* 102 (12): 1112–17.

Janvier, Annie, Barbara Farlow, and Keith J. Barrington. 2016. "Parental Hopes, Interventions, and Survival of Neonates with Trisomy 13 and Trisomy 18." *American Journal of Medical Genetics Part C: Seminars in Medical Genetics* 172 (3): 279–87.

Kittay, Eva Feder. 2009. "The Personal is Philosophical is Political: A Philosopher and Mother of a Cognitively Disabled Person Sends Notes from the Battlefield." *Metaphilosophy* 40 (3–4): 606–27.

Kosho, Tomoki, Hideo Kuniba, Yuko Tanikawa, Yoko Hashimoto, and Hiroko Sakurai. 2013. "Natural History and Parental Experience of Children with Trisomy 18 Based on a Questionnaire Given to a Japanese Trisomy 18 Parental Support Group." *American Journal of Medical Genetics Part A* 161 (7): 1531–42.

Kuebelbeck, Amy and Deborah L. Davis. 2011. *A Gift of Time: Continuing Your Pregnancy when your Baby's Life is Expected to be Brief.* Baltimore, MD: Johns Hopkins University Press.

Lahroodi, Reza. 2007. "Collective Epistemic Virtues." *Social Epistemology* 21 (3): 281–97.

Lakovschek, Ioana Claudia, Berthold Streubel, and Barbara Ulm. 2011. "Natural Outcome of Trisomy 13, Trisomy 18, and Triploidy after Prenatal Diagnosis." *American Journal of Medical Genetics Part A* 155 (11): 2626–33.

Leuthner, Steven R. 2004a. "Palliative Care of the Infant with Lethal Anomalies." *Pediatric Clinics of North America* 51 (3): 747–59.

Leuthner, Steven R. 2004b. "Fetal Palliative Care." *Clinics in Perinatology* 31 (3): 649–65.

Leuthner, Steven and Emilie Lamberg Jones. 2007. "Fetal Concerns Program: A Model for Perinatal Palliative Care." *MCN: The American Journal of Maternal/Child Nursing* 32 (5): 272–8.

MacIntyre, Alasdair C. 1999a. *Dependent Rational Animals: Why Human Beings Need the Virtues.* Chicago, IL: Open Court.

MacIntyre, Alasdair C. 1999b. "Social Structures and Their Threats to Moral Agency." *Philosophy* 74 (3): 311–29.

Marty, Colleen M. and Brian S. Carter. 2018. "Ethics and Palliative Care in the Perinatal World." *Seminars in Fetal and Neonatal Medicine* 23 (1): 35–8.

McCaffrey, Martin J. 2016. "Trisomy 13 and 18: Selecting the Road Previously Not Taken." *American Journal of Medical Genetics Part C: Seminars in Medical Genetics* 172 (3): 251–6.

Meyer, Robert E., Gang Liu, Suzanne M. Gilboa, Mary K. Ethen, Arthus S. Aylsworth, Cynthia M. Powell, Timothy J. Flood, Cara T. Mai, Ying Want, and Mark A. Canfield. 2016. "Survival of Children with Trisomy 13 and Trisomy 18: A Multi-State Population-Based Study." *American Journal of Medical Genetics Part A* 170 (4): 825–37.

Munson, David and Steven R. Leuthner. 2007. "Palliative Care for the Family Carrying a Fetus with a Life-limiting diagnosis." *Pediatric Clinics of North America* 54 (5): 787–98.

Norwitz, Errol R. and Brynn Levy. 2013. "Noninvasive Prenatal Testing: The Future is Now." *Reviews in Obstetrics & Gynecology* 6 (2): 48–62.

Parens, Erik and Adrienne Asch. 2000. *Prenatal Testing and Disability Rights.* Washington, DC: Georgetown University Press.

Poore, Gregory. 2014. "Why Care for the Severely Disabled? A Critique of MacIntyre's Account." *Journal of Medicine and Philosophy* 39 (4): 459–73.

Porpora, Douglas V. 1989. "Four Concepts of Social Structure." *Journal for the Theory of Social Behavior* 19 (2): 195–211.

Ramer-Chrastek, Joan and Megan V. Thygeson. 2005. "A Perinatal Hospice for an Unborn Child with a Life-limiting Condition." *International Journal of Palliative Nursing* 11 (6): 274–7.

Reinders, Hans. 2000. *The Future of the Disabled in Liberal Society*. Notre Dame: University of Notre Dame Press.

Roberts, Robert C. 1989. "Aristotle on Virtues and Emotions." *Philosophical Studies* 56 (3): 293–306.

Roush, Alana, Peggy Sullivan, Rhonda Cooper, and Judith W. McBride. 2007. "Perinatal Hospice." *Newborn and Infant Nursing Reviews* 7 (4): 216–21.

Sandelowski, Margarete and Julie Barroso. 2005. "The Travesty of Choosing after Positive Prenatal Diagnosis." *Journal of Obstetric, Gynecologic, & Neonatal Nursing* 34 (3): 307–18.

Sandelowski, Margarete and Linda Corson Jones. 1996. " 'Healing Fictions': Stories of Choosing in the Aftermath of the Detection of Fetal Anomalies." *Social Science & Medicine* 42 (3): 353–61.

Sandin, Per. 2007. "Collective Military Virtues." *Journal of Military Ethics* 6 (4): 303–14.

Schechtman, Kenneth B., Diana L. Gray, Jack D. Baty, and Steven M. Rothman. 2002. "Decision-Making for Termination of Pregnancies with Fetal Anomalies: Analysis of 53,000 Pregnancies." *Obstetrics & Gynecology* 99 (2): 216–22.

Schneiderman, Lawrence J., Nancy S. Jecker, and Albert R. Jonsen. 1990. "Medical Futility: Its Meaning and Ethical Implications." *Annals of Internal Medicine* 112 (12): 949–54.

Smith, Christian. 2010. *What is a Person? Rethinking Humanity, Social Life, and the Moral Good from the Person Up*. Chicago, IL: University of Chicago Press.

Smith, Michael D. 1982. "The Virtuous Organization." *Journal of Medicine and Philosophy* 7 (1): 31–42.

Snow, Nancy E. 2018. "Introduction." In *The Oxford Handbook of Virtue*, edited by Nancy E. Snow, 1–6. Oxford: Oxford University Press.

Sumner, Lizabeth H., Karen Kavanaugh, and Teresa Moro. 2006. "Extending Palliative Care into Pregnancy and the Immediate Newborn Period: State of the Practice of Perinatal Palliative Care." *The Journal of Perinatal & Neonatal Nursing* 20 (1): 113–16.

Toombs, S. Kay. 2018. *How Then Should We Die? Two Opposing Responses to the Challenges of Suffering and Death*. Elm Mott, TX: Colloquium Press.

Wasserman, David, Robert Wachbroit, and Jerome Bickenbach. 2005. *Quality of Life and Human Difference: Genetic Testing, Health Care, and Disability*. Cambridge: Cambridge University Press.

Watt, Helen. 2017. "Abortion for Life-Limiting Foetal Anomaly: Beneficial When and For Whom?" *Clinical Ethics* 12 (1): 1–10.

Whitfield, Jonathan M., Roberta Siegel, and Anita Glicken. 1982. "The Application of Hospice Concepts to Neonatal Care." *American Journal of Diseases of Children* 136 (5): 421–4.

Wilkinson, D.J.C., P. Thiele, A. Watkins, and L. Crespigny. 2012. "Authors' Response To: Fatally flawed?" *BJOG: An International Journal of Obstetrics & Gynaecology* 120 (11): 371–2.

Wilkinson, Dominic J.C. and Julian Savulescu. 2011. "Knowing When to Stop: Futility in the Intensive Care Unit." *Current Opinion in Anaesthesiology* 24 (2): 160–5.

Williams, Constance, David Munson, John Zupancic, and Haresh Kirpalani. 2008. "Supporting Bereaved Parents: Practical Steps in Providing Compassionate Perinatal and Neonatal End-of-life Care—A North American Perspective." *Seminars in Fetal and Neonatal Medicine* 13 (5): 335–40.

Williams, Constance. 2015. *Practical Virtues: An Evidence-Based Ethical Framework for Approaching End-of-Life Care in the Neonatal Intensive Care Unit.* PhD diss, University of Toronto.

Wool, Charlotte. 2011. "Systematic Review of the Literature: Parental Outcomes after Diagnosis of Fetal Anomaly." *Advances in Neonatal Care* 11 (3): 182–92.

Wool, Charlotte. 2013a. "State of the Science on Perinatal Palliative Care." *Journal of Obstetric, Gynecologic, & Neonatal Nursing* 42 (3): 372–82.

Wool, Charlotte. 2013b. "Clinician Confidence and Comfort in Providing Perinatal Palliative Care." *Journal of Obstetric, Gynecological & Neonatal Nursing* 42 (1): 48–58.

Yoon, John D., Kenneth A. Rasinski, and Farr A. Curlin. 2010. "Moral Controversy, Directive Counsel, and the Doctor's Role: Findings from a National Survey of Obstetrician-gynecologists." *Academic Medicine: Journal of the Association of American Medical Colleges* 85 (9): 1475–81.

Ziv, Anita Konzelmann. 2012. "Institutional Virtue: How Consensus Matters." *Philosophical Studies* 161 (1): 87–96.

2 Virtues of Acknowledged Dependence and Common Projects of Care

I. Introduction

Virtues are human excellences, characteristic expressions of moral and intellectual goodness in trait-relevant domains. Traditional discussions of virtues often focus on particular traits such as the cardinal virtues of courage, temperance, justice, and prudence. Each of these virtues is opposed by one or more vices—that is, settled traits that dispose a person to characteristic or habitual ways of missing the mark in the relevant domain. The vices of cowardice and rashness oppose courage; self-indulgence and insensibility oppose temperance; injustice opposes justice; and imprudence, negligence, and cleverness all oppose prudence.

Catalogs of virtues and opposing vices contain lists of dispositions beyond the cardinal virtues. Aristotle's expansive discussion of moral virtues in the central books of the *Nicomachean Ethics*, for instance, features no fewer than twelve individual virtues each flanked by opposing vices of excess and deficiency. Furthermore, he provides profiles of distinct intellectual virtues and describes the best form of friendship as a relationship rooted in a shared love of virtue.[1] Christian catalogs of the virtues include a range of unique dispositions including, perhaps most importantly, the theological virtues of faith, hope, and love. A range of vices opposes each of these virtues: resistant unbelief and heretical commitment oppose faith; despair and presumption oppose hope; hatred, sloth, and envy (among others) oppose charity. Canonical lists of Christian virtues also include character traits that act as remedies for the capital vices of pride, envy, wrath, greed, sloth, gluttony, and lust—respectively, these are the virtues of humility, kindness, patience, liberality, zeal, temperance, and chastity.[2] In the American context, Benjamin Franklin proposed a list of thirteen virtues: temperance, silence, order, resolution, frugality, industry, sincerity, justice, moderation, cleanliness, tranquility, chastity, and humility.[3] Contemporary philosophical discussions of the virtues and vices have extended the project of constructing profiles for specific virtues and their opposing vices.[4] Roberts and Wood (2007), for instance, seek to map a range of specifically intellectual character traits including (but not limited to): the love of knowledge, firmness, courage, caution, humility, autonomy, generosity, and practical wisdom. Other works in virtue epistemology focus on traits such as open-mindedness and epistemic self-vigilance.[5]

One striking feature of these varied catalogs is that they do not always feature the same dispositions. Depending on the list, one might find the specific traits construed as either a virtue or a vice. Humility offers the clearest illustration of this point. Christian theologians champion humility as a preeminent virtue, in part, because it acts as a corrective to the vice of pride.[6] Pride is a disposition that manifests itself variously in excessive concern for self-elevation and importance. According to one prominent strand of thought within the Christian tradition, pride is the ground of all the other vices—the ultimate corrupting source of human character.[7] It is not clear, however, that ancient Greek philosophers would characterize humility as a virtue or pride as a vice.[8] Likewise, the Early Modern philosopher David Hume expresses considerable skepticism about humility.[9] He contends that the 'monkish virtues' of humility, celibacy, fasting, penance, mortification, self-denial, silence, and solitude

> serve to no manner of purpose; neither advance a man's fortune in the world, nor render him a more valuable member of society; neither qualify him for the entertainment of company, nor increase his power of self-enjoyment . . . We observe, on the contrary, that they cross all these desirable ends; stupefy the understanding and harden the heart, obscure the fancy and sour the temper. We justly, therefore, transfer them to the opposite column, and place them in the catalogue of vices.
>
> (1995, 270)

Arguably, distinct catalogs of virtues and vices reflect diverging views of human nature and its ultimate good. Given differences in philosophical (and theological) anthropology, it is not clear that there will be a common or shared set of dispositions appearing on every catalog of canonical virtues.

Additionally, it is not clear that dispositions appearing on multiple lists admit of a univocal meaning. Consider, for instance, the virtue of courage. Courage is a virtue of proper self-management that enables one to remain committed to what one values in the midst of fearful or threatening circumstances. Robert Adams (2006) calls courage a *structural* rather than a *motivational* virtue because it lacks a specific moral concern of its own. Structural virtues are strengths of character that support commitment to and pursuit of other motivating concerns. Adams contends that they foster excellence in the ability and willingness "to govern one's life in accordance with one's own central aims and values, *whatever they are*" (2006, 37; emphasis added). But this generic definition may mask important differences in distinct analyses of courage—differences that become clear when one considers varied portraits of exemplary courage.

An account that points to the bravery of soldiers fighting on the bat-tlefield as the paradigmatic expression of courage differs in important respects from an account that points to the courage of martyrs willingly submitting to suffering and death.[10]

These complications affect both general theoretical discussion of the virtues and specific developments in applied virtue ethics. Thus, it is important to clarify my commitments at the outset of the work. Making these commitments explicit will also serve to distinguish my *virtue-based* defense from recent work that draws upon virtue-theoretic concepts. Constance Williams (2015) has developed a virtue-theoretic account that can be used to enhance end-of-life care in the NICU. Her study began as an attempt to understand distinct perspectives on the nature and quality of end-of-life care within this setting. In particular, she studied whether healthcare providers and families in the NICU shared goals and expec-tations concerning how to (i) understand quality end-of-life care and (ii) address uncertainties in the decision-making process. Furthermore, she sought to understand and address practical difficulties emerging from failures in communication and collaboration between and among various groups of healthcare providers engaged in the task of caring for affected families. Her virtue-theoretic framework sought to synthesize the varied perspectives represented in her research.

Williams contends that specific virtues facilitate quality communica-tion, decision-making, planning, and delivery of care in the NICU. She points to a long list of individual and collective traits that serve this aim including insightfulness, wisdom, thoughtfulness, courage, temperance, justice, honesty, integrity, trustworthiness, reliability, dependability, faith, hope, love, compassion, sympathy, empathy, loyalty, forgiveness, humility, attunement, openness, and responsiveness. As individual and collective traits, these virtues enable healthcare providers to address and resolve choice dilemmas emerging in difficult circumstances.

Both Williams and I endorse the view that virtue facilitates proper care for families within the NICU setting. We are both committed to the view that parents need healthcare providers and professional caregiving com-munities to exercise virtue in addressing both acknowledged and unrecog-nized needs. Furthermore, we agree that professional communities help to realize important goods through their commitment to and active engage-ment in structured and seamless care for the child and the family.[11] Many of her conclusions mirror conclusions I defend in the course of this book.

But my account differs from hers in several ways. First, Williams adopts a narrow definition of virtue fitting for her empirical methodol-ogy. She writes,

> a virtue is an essential trait of an individual [healthcare provider's] character or an essential trait attributed to an interprofessional team that enables them to navigate ethical dilemmas at [end-of-life]. When

practiced habitually, a virtue predisposes the [healthcare provider] and/or the interprofessional team to excellence of intent and performance with respect to the provision of good quality [end-of-life] care.

(2015, 36)

The virtue-theoretic framework she develops serves to systematize and explain the perspectives represented in a qualitative survey of clinicians and families in the NICU. By pointing to particular virtues, Williams shows how these traits could enhance quality end-of-life care for both families and clinicians. Williams rightly points to dispositions that are relevant in the NICU setting, but her framework is not rooted in a philosophical account of the nature and value of these traits independent of their exercise in the context of end-of-life dilemmas of care.

One may contrast this approach with my *virtue-based* defense which is grounded in a substantive philosophical commitment concerning the nature and value of specific human excellences. I frame my defense in terms of MacIntyre's (1999a) account of the virtues of acknowledged dependence. MacIntyre rightly notes the crucial connections between virtue and human vulnerability: part of what it means to possess and to exercise virtue is to be sensitive to and properly concerned for human needs. The virtues I describe in this work each take human vulnerabilities as focal objects of concern. I seek to map the contours of particular virtues that are responsive to these vulnerabilities.

Second, Williams rightly notes that families desire care from both individual healthcare providers and the full professional team charged with their care, but she does not provide a systematic philosophical framework that can justify her ascriptions of virtues to professional communities or medical institutions. My defense, however, offers an account sufficient to justify ascribing virtues (and opposing vices) to individuals, social groups, institutions, and social structures. Toward this end, I employ Robert Adams's (2006) account of common projects to show how individuals, personal communities, and institutions act together to address a family's need for care.[12] The team of healthcare providers and medical institutions who devote themselves to a caring participation in and support for these forms of care manifest virtue in response to profound human need.[13]

Third, Williams draws upon existing lists of virtues to show how specific traits are relevant for the provision of quality end-of-life care. She offers an extensive discussion of the ways particular virtues interact in the delivery of care, but she does not offer extended profiles of these forms of human excellence or their connection to important human goods. This is potentially problematic because the presence of a particular trait on a list of the virtues is not a guarantee that the trait is a virtue or, if it is, that there is a univocal conception of this virtue common to all lists. In this book, I offer extended profiles of virtues relevant to the particular needs of families. Developing substantive profiles of the sort serves to establish both the nature of the specific virtue and its status as a human excellence.

The aim of this chapter is to offer an extended discussion of the theoretical commitments central to my *virtue-based* defense. In Section II, I summarize MacIntyre's account of the virtues of acknowledged dependence, focusing on the vital role of local communities in fostering and sustaining these dispositions. In Section III, I propose that perinatal hospice is a good common project of care. Professional communities who commit to and care properly for this project manifest virtue. In Section IV, I contend that one may ascribe virtue to medical institutions if their social structures facilitate or safeguard caring commitment to a common project of care. In Section V, I conclude by suggesting that this *virtue-based* defense has important normative implications, especially for the reformation of deficient practices and social structures within contemporary care settings.

II. Vulnerability, Need, and Virtue

Alasdair MacIntyre is one of the few philosophers who places human vulnerability at the heart of moral discourse.[14] He writes,

> We human beings are vulnerable to many kinds of affliction and most of us are at some time afflicted by serious ills. How we cope is only in small part up to us. It is most often to others that we owe our survival, let alone our flourishing, as we encounter bodily illness and injury, inadequate nutrition, mental defect and disturbance, and human aggression and neglect. This dependence on particular others for protection and sustenance is most obvious in early childhood and in old age. But between these first and last stages our lives are characteristically marked by longer or short periods of injury, illness or other disablement and some among us are disabled for their entire lives. These two related sets of fact, those concerning our vulnerabilities and afflictions and those concerning the extent of our dependence on particular others are so evidently of singular importance that it might seem that no account of the human condition whose authors hoped to achieve credibility could avoid giving them a central place. Yet the history of Western moral philosophy suggests otherwise. From Plato to Moore and since there are usually, with some rare exceptions, only passing references to human vulnerability and affliction and to the connections between them and our dependence on others.
>
> (1999a, 1)

Seeking to redress this gap in the literature, MacIntyre offers an extended reflection on human vulnerability as a fundamental condition of our nature as dependent rational animals. A central element of his argument is an account of a distinct species of virtue—the virtues of acknowledged dependence. These virtues are dispositions of proper attunement to and vigilant care for human vulnerability both as a source of suffering and a ground of human fulfillment.[15] They dispose a person to fulfill the substantive moral task of caring for those whose conditions significantly diminish their prospects for flourishing. They also dispose him to appreciate his own needs and dependencies, inspiring in him a sense of indebtedness to others and gratitude for their concerned attention to his own vulnerabilities.

It is instructive in this context to consider MacIntyre's characterization of a particular virtue: *misericordia*.[16] MacIntyre construes *misericordia* as a virtue that disposes a person to characteristic patterns of merciful care for those who are suffering. The person who exercises *misericordia* tends to the needs of a person who is suffering. As a virtue, *misericordia* disposes a person to expressions of merciful care independent of natural bonds of friendship or communal attachment. The person with this virtue perceives need itself as a reason to respond. In fact, it is a mark of virtue that one is distressed by another's suffering and moved to respond independent of one's relation to the person. MacIntyre maintains that it is "the kind and scale of need that dictates what has to be done, not whose need it is" (1999a, 124). Put differently, *misericordia* involves mixed patterns of attention and inattention. The merciful person is attentive to suffering and experiences it as a summons to respond with care to the extent that he is able. He is inattentive to the sufferer's status as one *inside* or *outside* his community.

The exercise of *misericordia* makes it possible to form bonds with those who are initially outside the protection of one's community. Through this virtue, a community expands its boundaries to care for those in need as it would for its own members. One draws those who are vulnerable into the space of communal relationship in order to address their needs. MacIntyre writes,

> to direct the virtue of *misericordia* toward others is to extend one's communal relationships so as to include others within those relationships. And we are required from now on to care about them and to be concerned about their good just as we care about others already within our community.
>
> (1999a, 125–26)

In short, the person with the virtue of acknowledged dependence is disposed to address profound human needs, especially for those whose lives are marked by significantly life-limiting conditions. MacIntyre notes that those most likely to benefit from the wide distribution of these virtues within a community will be "those least capable of independent practical reasoning, the very young and the very old, the sick, the injured, and the otherwise disabled" (1999a, 108). Furthermore, he maintains that the flourishing of these individuals "will be an important index of the flourishing of the whole community. For it is insofar as it is *need* that provides reasons for action for the members of some particular community that that community flourishes" (1999a, 108–9).

This discussion illuminates crucial connections between interdependence and human fulfillment. First, interdependence is vital to the development of those virtues the exercise of which is necessary for a person to reason and to act well. MacIntyre notes that excellence in practical reasoning requires abilities (i) to appraise one's reasons for action, (ii) to detach oneself or stand back from occurrent desires that might undermine one's own or another's good, and (iii) to imagine distinct future possibilities that can orient one's actions. Cultivating these capacities is a precarious process complicated by common biological and social vulnerabilities. Fostering the dispositions necessary for excellent practical reasoning is much more likely within a community attuned to these vulnerabilities. A good community will help the individual to cultivate an attuned sensitivity to what is good along with the readiness to act in accordance with what is good. A good social environment supports the person in the cultivation and exercise of well-formed intellective and affective capacities— capacities that enable him to exercise the virtues crucial for living an excellent human life.[17] Thus, trusting dependence upon others is crucial for the ongoing development and exercise of virtues as an independent practical reasoner.

Second, and perhaps most importantly, proper forms of dependence enable one to forge, deepen, and extend relational bonds vital to human fulfillment.[18] Dependence is not something one must always overcome; it is not always a source of suffering. Consider, for instance, the ways love requires a willingness to embrace an inherent susceptibility to suffering. Willed vulnerability of this kind is crucial to the expression of love; it is fundamental to establishing and sustaining human relationships. Given that loving relationships are one of the chief goods of human life, embracing vulnerability is crucial to the cultivation of the relationships vital for a fulfilling human life.

If the proper embrace of human interdependence is a component of human flourishing, then individuals will flourish only to the extent that they are embedded within communities that are properly attentive and responsive to human vulnerability. Human flourishing is bound up in relationships of mutual giving and receiving—relationships in which "generally and characteristically, what and how far we are able to give depends in part on what and how far we received" (1999a, 99). The relationships that enable this kind of mutual giving and receiving are those constitutive of a local community.

MacIntyre conceives of a local community as a relatively small social group consisting of individuals, families, friends, neighbors, affiliations (e.g., a local church parish, colleagues), and other institutions and organizations that jointly work for the good of the community.[19]

On this view, neither the modern nation-state nor the family alone are properly described as local communities. The modern nation-state is too large, too diffuse, and too beholden to special interests jockeying for power to engage in the communal deliberation crucial to determining "how responsibilities for and to dependent others are allocated and what standards of success or failure in discharging these responsibilities are appropriate" (1999a, 133). This kind of deliberation requires intimate associations between and among members of local affiliations, networks of giving and receiving that enable members to join together in pursuit of a shared commitment to a common good for their community. Nation states can remove barriers or obstacles to human flourishing through significant actions (e.g., the passage of the Americans with Disabilities Act). But this is distinct from the kinds of tasks local communities fulfill in securing the common good for their members.

Families are key constituents within a local community, but the goods of the local community go beyond the goods of particular families.[20] MacIntyre writes,

> It is because of the family's lack of self-sufficiency that the type of common good recognition of which is required by the virtues of acknowledged dependence cannot be achieved within the family, at least insofar as the family is conceived of as a distinct and separate social unit.
>
> (1999a, 134–35)

Good families provide the primary ethos of social support for their children. But families are not the only ones with a responsibility to nurture the lives of their children. As I note elsewhere:

> Flourishing as a human being requires a network of social support beginning with the family and extending to friendships and other forms of local association. No family is sufficient unto itself for the development of virtue and the pursuit of the good.
>
> (Cobb 2016, 30)

What a family needs is an environment in which fulfilling a calling to love their children draws on the supportive care and resources of a broader community. In most cases, this will be a group characterized by deep and meaningful bonds of mutual support. One may construe the relations of support within a local community as structures of nested dependency.[21]

There are a number of implications one may draw from this discussion, but one point deserves emphasis: those communities who fail to inculcate and exercise virtues crucial to addressing human vulnerability are disproportionately bad for those whose needs are greatest.[22] Individuals with significantly life-limiting conditions and those most intimately involved in their care need communities disposed to meet their needs; their capacity for realizing human goods is radically dependent upon others. Those with the virtues of acknowledged dependence are disposed to fulfill these responsibilities. They are sensitive to and appreciative of both the gifts and the difficulties of human frailty. They attend properly to the vulnerabilities that ground significant moral tasks—tasks that cannot be addressed through the acts of individuals or families acting on their own. Whether, and the extent to which, a local community collectively tends to these needs is an important indicator of its excellence as a community.

I have devoted considerable space to summarizing MacIntyre's account of the virtues of acknowledged dependence because it serves as a central commitment in my defense of perinatal hospice. Individuals and communities who possess virtues of acknowledged dependence are disposed to respond well to the specific needs of families affected by an adverse *in utero* diagnosis. But my defense of perinatal hospice depends upon additional conceptual resources beyond MacIntyre's appeals to 'local communities' or 'networks of giving and receiving.' In particular, I draw upon Robert Adams's (2006) account of good common projects.[23]

There are three reasons I employ Adams's account in this context. First, perinatal hospice is a program of care targeting a fixed period of acute need: many of a family's needs following an adverse diagnosis occur in the time between diagnosis and the death of the child. Given these boundaries, the relations crucial for care are transient; they do not typically persist after the death of the child. These relationships are distinct from those that constitute the shared bonds within the family's personal community. The collective endeavor to provide for the family's need is better construed as a shared project involving the coordinated work of healthcare providers and institutions.

Second, individuals and institutions who address the needs of the family following a significantly life-limiting diagnosis typically interact with the family in fixed locations of care. The family has appointments with the obstetrician in a medical office; they meet with the care coordinator to construct a plan of care at the hospital; they deliver their child at a birthing center; the child receives care in the NICU; the chaplain meets with the family in the maternity ward to discuss their grief and help make plans for a funeral. The interactions between the family and those who provide perinatal hospice are typically bound to institutional spaces—spaces that automatically structure dynamics between caregivers and those who are in the position to receive care. The physical space that structures the family's experience in perinatal hospice is typically removed from those places in which they interact with their personal community. This spatial dislocation is another reason to distinguish the work of institutions and healthcare providers in providing perinatal hospice from the care a family's friends and family provide in their local communities.

Third, although personal communities can partly address a family's needs, there are dimensions of these needs that can only be addressed by healthcare providers and institutions. Perinatal hospice programs connect healthcare providers, professional communities, and medical institutions in a shared endeavor to support the family in their need. Through a coordinated and collaborative effort, varied actors fulfill institutional roles within a broad program of care. It is not healthcare providers acting alone; they act together within institutions that are structured, in part, to deliver care as part of a collective effort. Given the shared aims and the ways in which this project draws people and institutions together in a joint endeavor, it is fitting to think of perinatal hospice as a common project of care.

III. Virtue and Common Projects of Care

Robert Adams characterizes common projects as shared endeavors oriented around tasks, goals, and activities that are essentially social. Participating together as teammates, business partners, and colleagues; engaging in social roles and tasks such as parenting; the pursuit and development of friendships or other loving relationships—all of these projects join individuals together in a common or shared pursuit. We do few things in our lives separate from these kinds of joint pursuit.[24] As a result, many of the most important goods of human life are realized within the space of mutual participation in common projects. Adams contends that the

> human good is found very largely in activities whose point and value depend on the participation of other people in a common project. And the value of these activities depends on more than one person's caring about the common projects. Common projects are not mindless biological processes like digestion and metabolism. They exist only because people care about them. And if too many of the participants do not care enough about them, the activities connected with them are apt to lose value for all the participants.
>
> (2006, 88)

It is important to note that virtue does not manifest itself in an unqualified care for common projects. Virtue expresses itself in an apt care for *good* common projects. The virtuous person cares for the good and, thus, cannot care for bad common projects. It is not possible to care in an appropriate way for a project that is vicious. Engagement in bad common projects often contributes to the significant suffering of others. Thus, participating in these projects puts one in opposition to the good of others. As Adams observes,

> a vast amount of human involvement in evil is involvement in bad common projects. Probably the majority of the most horrendously evil projects are common projects of groups. In a bad common project, people will often perpetrate evils that few if any of them would choose if it were solely up to them.
>
> (2006, 86)

Caring for a bad common project is one of the ways participation in common projects can be flawed. But there are other forms of misplaced or inapt concern that affect one's participation in good common projects. The virtuous person's care for good common projects must be well-tuned.[25] To care properly for a good common project is to care in a way that is appropriate to the value of the project, to the ways it realizes important goods, and to its relative importance vis-à-vis other projects and goods. An individual's care should not be disproportionate to the value of the project; it should not display excessive or deficient devotion to the project; it should not distract him from weightier matters. Moreover, his care for the project should not express itself ruthlessly—that is, in actions or attitudes that disparage or devaluate other goods or persons. When one's care is apt, it demonstrates a proper orientation toward what is good: it orients one to the goods that are the object of the shared endeavor. A well-tuned concern for common projects is an excellent way of *being for* the good. It is also an excellent way of *being for* others—an allocentric orientation that is itself expressive of a central good of human life. Thus, Adams concludes that "a readiness to embrace good common projects for their own sake, and to participate in them loyally and well, is a virtue" (2006, 90). By implication, an unwillingness to commit to good common projects and the failure to participate in them with proper devotion and care are failures in virtue. One who fails to engage in these ways fails to orient himself both toward goods worth pursuing and toward others as proper subjects of moral concern.

I maintain that structured perinatal hospice programs are a kind of good common project. This is not to deny that professional communities may participate in these programs in a manner that fails to express virtue. But these programs characteristically orient professional communities and medical institutions toward important goods. An *apt* commitment to the practices characteristic of these programs combined with a collective endeavor to ensure their broad accessibility is a way of *being for* the good. These programs coordinate the efforts of individual healthcare providers, institutions of medical care, and personal communities to address the varied needs of a family in the midst of crisis. Providing this care involves integrating the efforts of a team of professionals including obstetricians, neonatologists, nurses, social workers, chaplains, counselors, and hospital administrators as well as the institutions that support and encourage this work. To care for the family effectively, all of these actors must engage in the effort to address the family's vulnerabilities. This joint endeavor reflects an allocentric orientation which is itself an expression of moral goodness.

Merely engaging in this project together, however, is not a guarantee that the individual healthcare providers or the institutions themselves are caring properly for this project. The actors must express a ready willingness to embrace and participate in this project with due diligence and care. For this reason, perinatal hospice programs as formal structures will not express or manifest virtue unless the actors who engage in these projects do so in a way that expresses a proper care both for the goods they promote and the individuals whose good they seek to secure. Caring properly for a good common project is virtuous because it expresses excellence in *being for* the good. An apt care for those in need and for those with whom one acts in service of these needs also expresses an excellence in being for others. Healthcare providers and institutions manifest virtue through this common project when their activities are accompanied by a proper care for both the project itself and the people whom the project serves. It is worth noting, however, that I typically employ the term 'perinatal hospice' as a shorthand for virtuous perinatal hospice programs—that is, those programs in which professional communities and medical institutions extend exemplary care. But the programs themselves without proper care and commitment from those engaged in caregiving are not sufficient for virtue.

Adams's account of good common projects provides a helpful resource to think about the ascription of virtue or vice to professional communities involved in the care of families affected by an adverse *in utero* diagnosis. One can ascribe virtue to those professional communities who devote themselves to promoting and providing perinatal hospice. Professional communities who fail to commit to this project or who display inadequate care or concern for affected families in their efforts fail to manifest virtue. Unfortunately, the burdens associated with this failure fall disproportionately on families who are already burdened by a devastating diagnosis and its meaning for their lives.

Failures to commit to or participate in this kind of project may be rooted in individual character flaws. But these failings may also be a function of inadequate structural support for individual healthcare providers or the professional community. The promotion and provision of virtuous forms of care often requires more than individual virtue; it requires a commitment from the institutions who support the efforts of the individual physicians, nurses, counselors, chaplains, and social workers who engage with the family. It requires social structures within these institutions that facilitate and safeguard caring commitment to this common project.[26]

IV. Institutions and Virtuous Social Structures

One of the central claims of this book is that one can ascribe virtue to institutions insofar as their social structures facilitate and safeguard a culture of caring commitment to the fulfillment of the project's aims.[27] Virtuous social structures enable healthcare providers and professional communities to identify, recognize, appreciate, and address particular vulnerabilities and needs. Institutions that fail to establish a culture of this sort fail to enact an important kind of institutional excellence. It does not follow from this that one should ascribe a vice to such an institution. There are multiple ways in which an institution may fail to express virtue without being vicious. But the failure to exercise virtue in care for these families is a failing that has adverse effects primarily on those who are most vulnerable.

It is instructive in this context to consider the nature and function of social structures in greater detail. In Chapter 1, I quoted the sociologist Christopher Smith (2010) in defining social structures as "durable systems of patterned social interaction" (322).[28] But Smith rightly acknowledges that this definition is overly general, offering in its place the following expanded definition:

> Social structures are: durable patterns of human social relations, generated and reproduced through social interactions and accumulated and transformed historically over time, that are expressed through lived bodily practices, which are defined by culturally meaningful cognitive categories, motivated in part by normative and moral valuations and guides, capacitated by and imprinted in material resources and artifacts, controlled and reinforced by regulative sanctions, which therefore promote cooperation and conformity and discourage resistance and opposition.
>
> (2010, 327)

The key components of this expanded definition help to illuminate (i) the ways social structures develop over time, (ii) how they frame interactions between and among individuals working within specific environments, (iii) the physical, social, and conceptual factors that contribute to their functional effects, and (iv) the conditions through which these structures become resistant to calls for reform. Social structures frame attitudes, expectations, roles, practices, protocols, and processes (among other factors). They establish a sense of normalcy and generate routine scripts that govern behavior within materially constrained environments. These framing conditions structure encounters between and among individuals within these spaces.[29]

I maintain that one can ascribe virtues to medical institutions insofar as their social structures encourage the exercise of virtue in response to the needs of families affected by an adverse *in utero* diagnosis. An institution that creates structures of support for this kind of work participates in a common project of care that realizes important goods. Institutions that fail to support this kind of work fail to manifest excellence in response to human needs. Consider, briefly, how social structures might inhibit or discourage active and caring commitment to the promotion and provision of perinatal hospice as a common project. Individual healthcare providers may find it difficult to care for families because the institutions in which they work fail to provide sufficient funding to provide such care. As a result, physicians who desire to provide such care may have to seek funding sources external to their institutions—a project that is too demanding given their available time and resources. Thus, an individually caring physician may be frustrated in his desire to promote and provide perinatal hospice because of an institutional unwillingness to fund such programs. Or, physicians may find their attempts to engage with the family in ways that are fitting for the family's needs frustrated by policies, procedures, or protocols that constrain their activities. Institutional protocols that restrict the amount of time physicians can spend with families can undercut the kind of caring concern crucial to addressing particular needs. Even if governing boards and individuals charged with leading these institutions seek to remedy these kinds of social structures, they may find their own attempts to promote and provide care frustrated by external social, economic, or legal barriers—obstacles that constrain the ways they can or must operate. These external social structures are often rooted in deeply entrenched social attitudes or political commitments that constrain the expected work of institutions. In short, the failure to provide proper care may be a consequence of deficient social structures rather than a failure in the virtues of individual healthcare providers or the team of healthcare professionals.[30]

One can extend this account by appealing to a distinction noted earlier between motivational and structural virtues. Recall that motivational virtues are dispositions rooted in a deep and abiding care or concern. Justice, for instance, is a disposition to care fundamentally about justice. The just person is disposed to act in pursuit of just institutions, just distribution of goods, and just social structures. He is pained by injustice and moved to seek remedy for the individual, communal, or political sources of this failure; he experiences joy when he sees that an individual has received what is proper to him or when an injustice has been rectified. Structural virtues, however, are not rooted in a specific motivating concern. Instead, they are virtues that enable one to pursue and remain committed to other moral concerns. Courage is a paradigmatic example of a structural virtue; it enables one to deal properly with threats of danger and fear such that one can remain oriented toward other moral goods. Courage acts to shore up the person's defenses so that he can pursue those things he loves even when this exposes him to fear and tempts him to recoil from these pursuits.

One may apply the distinction between motivational and structural virtues in the context of ascriptions of virtue to institutions. Some social structures orient the institution around particular moral concerns; other social structures enable institutions to manage threats or hindrances to the pursuit of important moral commitments. The former we might call institutionalized motivational virtues; the latter we can call institutionalized structural virtues. Applied to perinatal hospice programs, I contend that those social structures that promote an allocentric concern for affected families are institutionalized motivational virtues. Those social structures that enable institutions to manage those factors that threaten institutional participation in or commitment to this common project of care might be construed as institutionalized structural virtues.

One can summarize the basic argument of this section thus: some types of social structures encourage or facilitate participation in good common projects either by promoting an internal concern for particular goods or by facilitating strengths of collective will to counter or manage those factors that may inhibit the pursuit of important goods. Other social structures, however, fail to promote virtue either by failing to foster other-regarding moral concern or by failing to create structural defenses that can safeguard the pursuit of significant goods. These deficient structures can inhibit individual and institutional engagement with and concern for families affected by adverse *in utero* diagnoses. They can discourage the proper participation in a common project of care. Moreover, individuals who act in accordance with these structures may not realize how their actions and attitudes compound the difficulties of those who are profoundly vulnerable.[31] At a further extreme, some social structures may promote the expression of vice. Individuals who act in accordance with these vicious social structures may fail to recognize their complicity in the promotion of a vicious culture.

Perinatal hospice programs depend upon the joint participation of individual healthcare providers and the institutions in which they work. Unfortunately, there is evidence that families experience deficient care at the individual and institutional level. Addressing failures of particular individual healthcare providers may alleviate some of the harms these families face. But the exercise of virtue by individual healthcare providers may not address the full range of needs. These physicians and nurses may find their work particularly difficult within systems that inhibit caring concern for these families. For institutions that lack virtuous social structures, structural remedies may be necessary. As Elizabeth Anderson (2012) notes, "Many structural remedies are in place to enable individual virtue to work, by giving it favorable conditions" (168).[32] The careful articulation of an account of virtuous social structures can help to identify the types of structural reform crucial for realizing moral goods. It is this kind of structural remedy that can facilitate better forms of care for families who receive an adverse *in utero* diagnosis.

V. Conclusion—Needs, Virtues, and Perinatal Hospice

Perinatal hospice is a common project of care that addresses important human needs in the midst of great difficulty. It manifests important virtues as it tends to profound human needs rooted in common vulnerabilities. In the next few chapters, I describe four virtues that take particular needs and vulnerabilities as focal objects of concern. Three of these virtues are best construed as *motivational* virtues—that is, they are virtues rooted in an orienting concern for particular moral goods. Hospitality, solidarity, and compassion are each grounded in a caring concern for the wellbeing of others. They are natural members of a cluster of allocentric virtues. As I noted in Chapter 1, the fourth virtue, hope, is not a *motivational* virtue. It is better construed as an emotion-virtue—that is, a disposition for well-tuned affective appraisal of goods that are possible but difficult to secure. Hopes for or on another's behalf, however, can be an expression of the virtue of hope rooted in allocentric concern. Thus, allocentric hope can be included within the cluster of virtues I describe in this work as crucial to addressing the needs of families affected by an adverse *in utero* diagnosis.

A crucial feature of my defense is ascription of virtues or vices to professional communities of healthcare providers and medical institutions. I have suggested that professional communities manifest virtue to the extent that they commit to a caring engagement in a common project that addresses human needs and vulnerabilities. Thus, professional communities express virtue through their commitment to promoting and providing perinatal hospice. One can ascribe virtue to medical institutions to the extent that their social structures facilitate or safeguard proper care and commitment to this common project of concern. In the following chapters, I describe social structures that exhibit hospitality, allocentric hope, solidarity, and compassion. Given that the cluster of allocentric virtues I have identified share a substantive moral concern for the wellbeing of families, these institutionalized virtues orient individuals and groups around an expression of moral concern for affected families. By acting in accordance with these structures, individual healthcare providers and the caregiving team express virtuous care in addressing a family's needs.

My *virtue-based* defense has important normative implications for medical practice. It is worth highlighting some of these implications here, reserving the full discussion for later chapters. The virtue of hospitality enjoins physicians, nurses, and others involved in the family's care to reframe the language they employ in discussing the child, his condition, and his prognosis. Furthermore, it summons them to reframe their counseling practices such that the family feels invited into a space of care. The virtuous expression of allocentric hope can lead professional communities to extend a vision of the kinds of goods families can realize even if curative and therapeutic practices will not alter the difficult realities they face. This kind of hopeful vision can help families to recover a sense of the meaningfulness of carrying the pregnancy to term. The virtue of solidarity moves healthcare providers and institutions to be present to the family in the midst of their wait for birth and death. Walking with the family in this way involves coordinating care, developing contingency plans for various outcomes, working across institutional spaces to ensure that they do not experience fragmentation in care, and ensuring that they are embedded within social support groups if needed. Finally, the virtue of compassion can move professional communities and medical institutions to attend well to the wide range of losses families experience, offering consolation for both anticipatory and present griefs. This compassionate engagement may involve embracing a more demanding conception of care than is currently in practice. It calls physicians, nurses, chaplains, and social workers to an attuned and engaged willingness to suffer with the family.

In short, my *virtue-based* defense implies that individuals, professional communities, and institutions display excellence through their commitment to promote and provide perinatal hospice. Virtuous communities respond to the needs of families by devoting resources to ensure the wide availability of these programs. They gladly take on needed reforms to social structures and routine practices such that affected families can readily access these forms of care. Those communities who fail to respond to this call may not be vicious, but they will likely compound the burdens of affected families. Individuals, professional communities, and medical institutions who are sensitive to virtue will be moved to enact reforms to care for families and their unmet needs.

Notes

1 On this point, see Alfano (2016).
2 In addition to this, Christian theological accounts of the moral life include discussions of the gifts and fruit of the Holy Spirit as well as the beatitudes. For discussion of these distinctive dimensions of Christian virtue theory, see Pinsent (2012).
3 Under each of these virtues, Franklin lists a particular precept that specifies the behaviors and attitudes it enjoins. Under industry, for instance, he writes, "Lose no time; be always employ'd in something useful; cut off all unnecessary actions" (1916, 148). Commenting on this particular virtue, Alasdair MacIntyre (1981) observes that Franklin

> clearly considers the drive to acquire itself a part of virtue, whereas for most ancient Greeks this is the vice of *pleonexia*; [Franklin] treats some virtues which earlier ages had considered minor as major; but he also redefined familiar virtues. In the list of thirteen virtues which Franklin compiled as part of his system of private moral accounting, he elucidates each virtue by citing a maxim, obedience to which *is* the virtue in question. In the case of chastity the maxim is 'Rarely use venery but for health or offspring—never to dullness, weakness or the injury of your own or

another's peace or reputation'. This is clearly not what earlier writers had meant by 'chastity'.

(28)

4 Timpe and Boyd (2014) provide a wide-ranging collection of essays on individual virtues and opposing vices.

5 For discussions, see Baehr (2011) and Roberts and West (2015). Some recent work focuses on developing profiles of intellectual vices. See Baehr (2010); Battaly (2010, 2014); and Cassam (2016).

6 See Boyd (2014). Dunnington (2019) argues that no contemporary secular or religious account of humility adequately characterizes early Christian conceptions of humility.

7 See DeYoung (2007).

8 In this context, it is helpful to contrast Aristotelian and Thomistic accounts of the virtue of magnanimity. For helpful discussion, see DeYoung (2004); Herdt (2008); and MacIntyre (1999a).

9 For some recent discussion of Hume's view on "monkish virtues," see Button (2005) and Reed (2012).

10 See DeYoung (2012) for an instructive comparison of the warrior and the martyr as exemplars of courage. The heroic courage of the warrior requires strengths of body and mind that enable the person to act aggressively against threats in order to preserve the goods for which he fights. The courage required of the martyr is a strength born of the realization that one cannot avoid or defeat ultimate threats; instead, one must face the threat and accept its power to destroy one's life. This is a strength of soul that accepts the inevitable reality of death because willing submission is the only way to exercise one's commitment to the good.

11 Williams's (2015) analysis points to some very important concerns that deserve greater attention than I can provide here. In particular, her focus on the moral distress of healthcare providers resulting from either family choices or the difficulties within the caregiving team is particularly relevant to the social structures crucial to providing quality care. Furthermore, the discussion of the moral residue of choices at the end of life is particularly important for thinking through the difficulties and burdens for both the family and the caregivers. I return to some of these issues in Chapter 7.

12 Camenisch (2001, 239) distinguishes between (i) personal communities of friends, family, and local affiliations such as local churches and (ii) professional or functional communities of healthcare providers and institutions. I follow Camenisch in using the term 'professional community' to refer to those individuals and institutions that are involved in caring for the family within institutional spaces.

13 For recent defenses of the ascription of virtues and vices to collective or groups, see Anderson (2012); Beggs (2003); Byerly and Byerly (2016); Fricker (2010); Lahroodi (2007); Sandin (2007); Smith (1982); and Ziv (2012).

14 When affliction and dependence is a subject of concern for moral philosophers, they tend to focus on vulnerable individuals as passive recipients of care. This approach seems to presuppose that the vulnerable are fundamentally different from those who are delivering care. MacIntyre asserts that this approach fails to appreciate the ways in which both the caregiver and the recipient are alike—both are susceptible to common vulnerabilities.

15 For helpful discussions of MacIntyre's account, see Boyd (2014); Dunne (2002); and Poore (2014).

16 Traditionally, theologians have characterized *misericordia* as an extension of the theological virtue of *caritas*—a disposition of love for God and all God

loves. MacIntyre refers specifically to St. Thomas Aquinas who defines *misericordia,* or mercy, as the "heartfelt sympathy for another's distress, impelling us to succor him if we can. For mercy takes its name *'misericordia'* from denoting a man's compassionate heart [*miserum cor*] for another's unhappiness" (Aquinas 1948, 1311). But MacIntyre contends that *misericordia* deserves "its place in the catalogue of the virtues, independently of its theological grounding" (1999a, 124). He argues that the kind of love expressed through *misericordia* (i) is recognized as a virtue by nonreligious philosophical authorities and (ii) is "recognizably at work in the secular world" (124). Poore (2014) offers an extended critique of MacIntyre's attempts to develop a theologically neutral account of the virtue of *misericordia*. For further discussion of *misericordia,* see Miner (2015); O'Callaghan (2015); and Ryan (2010).

17 MacIntyre's extensive discussions of virtue have consistently emphasized the importance of community in moral formation. In *After Virtue* (2007), community is central to his notion of practices, his understanding of the narrative unity of a life, his account of the role of traditions in sustaining and transmitting practices and various forms of life, and, most importantly, his articulation of the need for the virtues. MacIntyre (1984) also outlines a number of ways community is central to a person's moral commitments. Lawrence Blum's (1994) work on the connections between moral identity, community, and virtue is indebted to MacIntyre's early works.

18 For additional discussion of human need as a source of vulnerability and fulfillment, see Wolfe 2016.

19 For a sympathetic discussion of the need for local associations who can provide for the needs of those with disabilities, see Reinders (2000). For important critical engagement with MacIntyre on the nature of local communities, see Dunne (2002); Hibbs (2004); and Murphy (2003).

20 For critical engagement with MacIntyre's account of the family, see Bishop (2015).

21 See Kittay (1999, 2011) for further discussion.

22 Poore (2014) argues that MacIntyre's account fails to show we ought to care for individuals with profound disabilities who are not already members of a local community. Unfortunately, I lack the space to consider this critique.

23 Arguably, the account I offer in what follows is one way of specifying what it is to be a 'local community' or 'network of giving and receiving.' Those individuals, groups, and institutional actors who participate well in a common project of care for families may be characterized as a type of local community which enacts a network of giving and receiving.

24 For related discussion, see Baier (1997) and Sherman (1993).

25 For discussion of some difficulties in interpreting Adams's account of virtue as an excellence in being for the good, see Poore (2011).

26 In many ways, this discussion connects with important themes from MacIntyre's earlier works. In *After Virtue*, MacIntyre (2007) discusses relations between institutions, practices, and the virtues. Institutions have an important role to play in the sustaining practices vital to the realization of common goods within a given social context. But they are oriented largely toward the acquisition and promotion of external goods—especially economic goods. For this reason, institutions can fulfill their role in sustaining good social practices only to the extent that the institution itself does not give itself over to the corrupting pull of the pursuit of external goods. The creation and maintenance of institutions that serve the common good requires dispositions and practices of resistance to an over-valuation of external goods. Thus, the virtues are necessary to protect a practice from the corrupting power of institutions. Likewise, MacIntyre (1999b) discusses the ways in which some social structures can threaten the exercise of moral agency.

27 My aim is to offer an account sufficient for the ascription of virtue (or vice) to institutional and social structures. There is a growing body of literature defending the view that there are collective or group virtues, but it is not essential to my discussion that I endorse this view. For helpful discussions of these debates see Byerly and Byerly (2016) and Cordell (2016).

28 For an analysis of distinct account of social structures, see Porpora (1989).

29 For further discussion, see Haslanger (2012, 413–18).

30 I return to these issues and address them at much greater length in Chapter 7.

31 Adams and Balfour (2009) develop an account of administrative evil, according to which

> ordinary people may simply be acting appropriately in their organizational role—in essence, just doing what those around them would agree they should be doing—and at the same time, participating in what a critical and reasonable observer, usually well after the fact, would call *evil*. Even worse . . . ordinary people can all too easily engage in acts of administrative evil while believing that what they are doing is not only correct, but in fact, good.
>
> (4)

32 Anderson contends that structural remedies are "virtue-based remedies for collective agents" (2012, 168).

References

Adams, Guy B. and Danny L. Balfour. 2009. *Unmasking Administrative Evil*. 3rd Edition. Armonk, NY: M.E. Sharpe.

Adams, Robert. 2006. *A Theory of Virtue: Excellence in Being for the Good*. Oxford: Clarendon Press.

Alfano, Mark. 2016. "Friendship and the Structure of Trust." In *From Personality to Virtue: Essays on the Philosophy of Character*, edited by Alberto Masala and Jonathan Webber, 186–206. Oxford: Oxford University Press.

Anderson, Elizabeth. 2012. "Epistemic Justice as a Virtue of Social Institutions." *Social Epistemology* 26 (2): 163–73.

Aquinas, Thomas. 1948. *The Summa Theologica of St. Thomas Aquinas*. Notre Dame, IN: Christian Classics.

Baehr, Jason S. 2010. "Epistemic Malevolence." In *Virtue and Vice, Moral and Epistemic*, edited by Heather Battaly, 189–213. Malden, MA: Wiley-Blackwell.

Baehr, Jason S. 2011. *The Inquiring Mind: On Intellectual Virtues and Virtue Epistemology*. Oxford: Oxford University Press.

Baier, Annette. 1997. "Doing Things with Others: The Mental Commons." In *Commonality and Particularity in Ethics*, edited by Lilli Alanen, Sara Heinämaa, and Thomas Wallgren, 15–44. Palgrave Macmillan.

Battaly, Heather. 2010. "Epistemic Self-Indulgence." In *Virtue and Vice, Moral and Epistemic*, edited by Heather Battaly, 215–30. Malden, MA: Wiley-Blackwell.

Battaly, Heather. 2014. "Varieties of Epistemic Vice." In *The Ethics of Belief: Individual and Social*, edited by Jonathan Matheson and Rico Vitz, 51–76. Oxford: Oxford University Press.

Beggs, Donald. 2003. "The Idea of Group Moral Virtue." *Journal of Social Philosophy* 34 (3): 457–74.

Bishop, Jeffrey. 2015. "Dependency, Decisions, and a Family of Care." In *Family-Oriented Informed Consent*, edited by Ruiping Fan, 27–42. Dordrecht: Springer International Publishing.

Blum, Lawrence A. 1994. *Moral Perception and Particularity*. Cambridge: Cambridge University Press.

Boyd, Craig A. 2014. "Pride and Humility: Tempering the Desire for Excellence." In *Virtues and Their Vices*, edited by Kevin Timpe and Craig A. Boyd, 245–68. Oxford: Oxford University Press.

Button, Mark. 2005. "'A Monkish Kind of Virtue'? For and Against Humility." *Political Theory* 33 (6): 840–68.

Byerly, T. Ryan and Meghan Byerly. 2016. "Collective Virtue." *The Journal of Value Inquiry* 50 (1): 33–50.

Camenisch, Paul F. 2001. "Communities of Care, of Trust, and of Healing." In *Medicine and the Ethics of Care*, edited by Diana Fritz Cates and Paul Lauritzen, 234–69. Washington, DC: Georgetown University Press.

Cassam, Quassim. 2016. "Vice Epistemology." *The Monist* 99 (2): 159–80.

Cobb, Aaron D. 2016. "Acknowledged Dependence and the Virtues of Perinatal Hospice." *Journal of Medicine and Philosophy* 41 (1): 25–40.

Cordell, Sean. 2016. "Group Virtues: No Great Leap Forward with Collectivism." *Res Publica* 23 (1): 43–59.

DeYoung, Rebecca Konyndyk. 2004. "Aquinas's Virtues of Acknowledge Dependence: A New Measure of Greatness," *Faith and Philosophy* 21 (2): 214–27.

DeYoung, Rebecca Konyndyk. 2007. *Glittering Vices: A New Look at the Seven Deadly Sins and Their Remedies*. Grand Rapids, MI: Brazos Press.

DeYoung, Rebecca Konyndyk. 2012. "Courage." In *Being Good: Christian Virtues for Everyday Life*, edited by Michael W. Austin and R. Douglas Geivett, 145–66. Grand Rapids, MI: Wm. B. Eerdmans Publishing Company.

Dunne, Joseph. 2002. "Ethics Revised: Flourishing as Vulnerable and Dependent. A Critical Notice of Alasdair MacIntyre's *Dependent Rational Animals*." *International Journal of Philosophical Studies* 10 (3): 339–63.

Dunnington, Kent. 2019. *Humility, Pride and Christian Virtue Theory*. Oxford: Oxford University Press.

Franklin, Benjamin. 1916. *Autobiography of Benjamin Franklin*, ed. F.W. Pine. New York: Henry Holt and Company.

Fricker, Miranda. 2010. "Can There Be Institutional Virtues?" In *Oxford Studies in Epistemology, Social Epistemology*, edited by Tamar Szabo Gendler and John Hawthorne, 235–52. Oxford: Oxford University Press.

Haslanger, Sally. 2012. *Resisting Reality: Social Construction and Social Critique*. Oxford: Oxford University Press.

Herdt, Jennifer. 2008. *Putting on Virtue: The Legacy of the Splendid Vices*. Chicago, IL: University of Chicago Press.

Hibbs, Thomas. S. 2004. "MacIntyre, Aquinas, and Politics." *The Review of Politics* 66 (3): 357–83.

Hume, David. 1995. *Enquiries Concerning Human Understanding and Concerning the Principles of Morals*. Oxford: Clarendon Press.

Kittay, Eva Feder. 1999. *Love's Labor: Essays on Women, Equality and Dependency*. London: Routledge.

Kittay, Eva Feder. 2011. "The Ethics of Care, Dependence, and Disability." *Ratio Juris* 24 (1): 49–58.

Lahroodi, Reza. 2007. "Collective Epistemic Virtues." *Social Epistemology* 21 (3): 281–97.

MacIntyre, Alasdair C. 1984. "Is Patriotism a Virtue?" *The Lindley Lecture.* Lawrence, KS: University of Kansas.

MacIntyre, Alasdair C. 1999a. *Dependent Rational Animals: Why Human Beings Need the Virtues.* Chicago, IL: Open Court.

MacIntyre, Alasdair C. 1999b. "Social Structures and Their Threats to Moral Agency." *Philosophy* 74 (3): 311–29.

MacIntyre, Alasdair C. 2007. *After Virtue.* 3rd Edition. Notre Dame: University of Notre Dame Press.

MacIntyre, Alasdair. 1981. "The Nature of the Virtues." *Hastings Center Report* 11 (2): 27–34.

Miner, Robert. 2015. "The Difficulties of Mercy: Reading Thomas Aquinas on Misericordia." *Studies in Christian Ethics* 28 (1): 70–85.

Murphy, Mark. 2003. "MacIntyre's Political Philosophy." In *Alasdair MacIntyre: Contemporary Philosophy in Focus,* edited by Mark C. Murphy, 152–75. Cambridge: Cambridge University Press.

O'Callaghan, John. 2015. "*Misericordia* in Aquinas: A Test Case for Theological and Natural Virtues." In *Faith, Hope, and Love: Thomas Aquinas on Living by the Theological Virtues,* edited by Harm Goris, Lambert Hendriks, and Henk Schoot, 215–32. Leuven: Peeters.

Pinsent, Andrew. 2012. *The Second-Person Perspective in Aquinas's Ethics: Virtues and Gifts.* London: Routledge.

Poore, Gregory. 2011. "Reconciling Robert Adams' Accounts of Virtues and Motivational Virtues." *Southwest Philosophy Review* 27 (2): 123–40.

Poore, Gregory. 2014. "Why Care for the Severely Disabled? A Critique of MacIntyre's Account." *Journal of Medicine and Philosophy* 39 (4): 459–73.

Porpora, Douglas V. 1989. "Four Concepts of Social Structure." *Journal for the Theory of Social Behavior* 19 (2): 195–211.

Reed, Philip. 2012. "What's Wrong with Monkish Virtues? Hume on the Standard of Virtue." *History of Philosophy Quarterly* 29 (1): 39–56.

Reinders, Hans. 2000. *The Future of the Disabled in Liberal Society.* Notre Dame: University of Notre Dame Press.

Roberts, Robert C. and Ryan West. 2015. "Natural Epistemic Defects and Corrective Virtues." *Synthese* 192 (8): 2557–76.

Roberts, Robert C. and W. Jay Wood. 2007. *Intellectual Virtues: An Essay in Regulative Epistemology.* Oxford: Oxford University Press.

Ryan, Thomas. 2010. "Aquinas on Compassion: Has He Something to Offer Today?" *Irish Theological Quarterly* 75 (2): 157–74.

Sandin, Per. 2007. "Collective Military Virtues." *Journal of Military Ethics* 6 (4): 303–14.

Sherman, Nancy. 1993. "The Virtues of Common Pursuit." *Philosophy and Phenomenological Research* 53 (2): 277–99.

Smith, Christian. 2010. *What is a Person? Rethinking Humanity, Social Life, and the Moral Good from the Person Up.* Chicago, IL: University of Chicago Press.

Smith, Michael D. 1982. "The Virtuous Organization." *Journal of Medicine and Philosophy* 7 (1): 31–42.

Timpe, Kevin and Craig A. Boyd. 2014. *Virtues and Their Vices.* Oxford: Oxford University Press.

Williams, Constance. 2015. *Practical Virtues: An Evidence-Based Ethical Framework for Approaching End-of-Life Care in the Neonatal Intensive Care Unit.* PhD diss, University of Toronto.

Wolfe, Katherine. 2016. "Together in Need: Relational Selfhood, Vulnerability to Harm, and Enriching Attachments." *Southern Journal of Philosophy* 54 (1): 129–48.

Ziv, Anita Konzelmann. 2012. "Institutional Virtue: How Consensus Matters." *Philosophical Studies* 161 (1): 87–96.

3 Life-Limiting Diagnoses and the Virtue of Hospitality

I. Introduction

One of the immediate needs parents experience following an adverse *in utero* diagnosis is the need to be received into a space of care. But they often confront unwelcoming attitudes, practices, and social structures that compound the difficulties of their experience. In some cases, healthcare providers and institutions act with apparent hostility toward the decision to continue an affected pregnancy.[1]

Consider a particularly vivid case. At a routine prenatal scan, Siri Berg and Odd Paulsen learned that their unborn daughter, Evy, had trisomy 18. Their geneticist immediately suggested that they should terminate the pregnancy, but they declined this offer because they "loved this baby, had seen its heart beat, its legs kick, and studied its beautiful profile" (Berg, Paulsen, and Carter 2013, 406). Confused by the decision, the geneticist objected: "Everybody chooses abortion" (Berg, Paulsen, and Carter 2013, 406). Similarly, their obstetrician openly challenged their choice, urging them to consider the burdens Evy's life and death would cause for their four other children. She assured them there was no point in continuing the pregnancy because trisomy 18 was " 'incompatible with life,' 'lethal,' a condition filled with unbearable suffering" (Berg, Paulsen, and Carter 2013, 406).[2] She promised them that they would "soon begin to wish that it dies in utero" (Berg, Paulsen, and Carter 2013, 406).

As the pregnancy continued, they faced additional barriers to care. Ultrasound technicians displayed a lack of sensitivity to their unique circumstances. When conducting routine tests, they failed to acknowledge the diagnosis and, at times, failed to demonstrate respect for Evy as a dearly loved child. Additionally, consultations with physicians at a local birthing center revealed that children with trisomy 18 were not monitored during delivery—a departure from routine practice. A neonatologist informed them that he would not perform any interventions after birth because these were merely "a means to postpone death" and "there was nothing that could be done for these 'lethal babies' " (Berg, Paulsen, and Carter 2013, 406). Berg and Paulsen write,

> The physician gave us the impression that this monster should have been removed long ago and that she was as good as dead. All treatments, including palliation, were to be avoided. Neonates with trisomy 18 were, apparently, to be left to die, sooner rather than later.
> (Berg, Paulsen, and Carter 2013, 406–7)

They eventually found a hospital willing to offer minimal support measures at birth. But upon delivery, the attending physician refused to provide positive pressure ventilation—an intervention which he agreed to perform prior to delivery. So, against the wishes of the healthcare providers, Paulsen, a trained anesthetist, took matters into his own hands, providing oxygen support through bag ventilation. Reflecting on their experience as a whole, Berg writes:

> Why were they in such a hurry to see her die? She did not suffer, we would not allow that. Her siblings got time to hold her, love her, and create memories. We were a whole family for this short time. The initial bagging/mask ventilation performed by my husband's actions gave us [three] beautiful days with Evy Kristine instead of just minutes; time that is of infinite value in a life presumed to be short. On her third day of life her heart got weaker. We knew the end was near. She now seemed bothered by the CPAP so we removed it. She died peacefully in my arms [five] hours later. We knew her life would be short and we regarded every minute with her as a gift. She taught us so much in her short life; for, surely, even a life of [three] days is a life. Our family is richer for it. Assuredly that is worth something.
> (Berg, Paulsen, and Carter 2013, 407)

Berg and Paulsen's experience falls on the extreme end of a spectrum of regrettably common encounters following an adverse *in utero* diagnosis. Health care professionals often frame a family's options in ways that imply continuing the pregnancy is pointless or cruel.[3] The language they employ to describe the child or his condition can cast doubt upon the child's value and invalidate a mother or father's sense of parental identity. Physicians may fail to demonstrate sufficient sensitivity to prognostic uncertainty; their language about the potential for suffering may be insufficiently circumspect. Additionally, healthcare providers and institutions may fail to describe or offer support for alternative forms of care.[4] They may fail to articulate the kinds of goods that can be realized through comfort-maximizing practices. Medical institutions that have the capacity to provide this support may fail to make these modalities of care readily accessible.

In this chapter, I contrast these practices and social structures with the welcome made available through the promotion and provision of perinatal hospice. The central aim of this discussion is to show how perinatal hospice programs manifest the virtue of hospitality. In Section II, I summarize evidence indicating that families experience unwelcoming encounters following an adverse diagnosis. In Section III, I develop an account of the individual virtue of hospitality, contrasting it with various species of vicious inhospitality and other forms of deficient welcome. In Section IV, I show how professional communities and institutions manifest hospitality through a common project of welcoming whole families and their unborn children into a space of protection and care. I contend that social structures within these institutions are hospitable to the extent that they facilitate or safeguard caring participation in this common endeavor. In this section, I provide a concrete illustration of the nature and expression of hospitality within professional communities and institutions. Finally, in Section V, I conclude by describing some practical steps toward fostering an institutional culture more hospitable to families who have received an adverse *in utero* diagnosis.

II. Life-Limiting Diagnoses and the Need for Welcome

There is a growing body of literature on the difficulties families experience in securing care for their children following an adverse *in utero* diagnosis. This is perhaps most clear in reports of the pressures to terminate affected pregnancies. In some cases, this pressure is overt. In a recent study of 332 families of children diagnosed with trisomy 13 or 18, Guon et al. (2014) note that a majority of these families (61%) felt pressure to terminate the pregnancy. One of the participants in the survey noted that a geneticist informed her that "the only way [she] could get an appointment with the main Obstetrician was if [she] was booking in for a termination" (312). Another reported that her obstetrician "encouraged abortion, saying that we would never find any doctors to treat her. We would be doing her a favor by saving her from suffering" (312). One couple was told that "abortion was definitely the best option for us and [we] had full support to have an abortion right up until my [twenty-sixth] week of pregnancy" (312). Other parents were told that "if they terminated their pregnancy, they could 'go on with their life' or 'have another child'" (314). Another family who refused the offer to terminate the pregnancy was told that "the best thing that can happen now is if your baby dies then you can get over this and try again" (312).[5]

In many cases, however, the pressure is subtle, arising from the ways physicians and genetic counselors frame the family's choices. Consider, for instance, the simple statement that most families in these circumstances choose to terminate the pregnancy. When a person with medical authority states that termination is typical, a family may think that the choice to continue a pregnancy requires defying a norm. Expressed reservations concerning or a refusal to comply with this norm may elicit reactions of surprise, confusion, or even anger. And there are other potentially biasing framing effects. Physicians may use language that is value-laden to suggest that there is no reason to continue the pregnancy. Or, their prognoses may not be sufficiently sensitive to new evidence concerning longevity or to the efficacy of more aggressive interventions. They may fail to exercise sufficient caution in their statements concerning the child's condition and the potential for suffering. Furthermore, there are usually pressures on the family's decision emerging from the need to make a quick decision. Given the regulations governing the practice of abortion, physicians may urge families to deliberate quickly in order to ensure that they can exercise their legal rights to terminate the pregnancy.[6] If they fail to mention or discuss alternative modalities of care, families may be left with a sense that there are no other live options. They may resign themselves to the view that continuing an affected pregnancy is not a real or genuinely meaningful possibility. These are just a few of the ways physicians frame choice options that may be construed as a begrudging willingness to provide care.

There are several recent studies that offer evidence of these kinds of subtle pressures. In one study, Farrelly et al. (2012) note that genetic counselors mentioned pregnancy termination in 86% of cases following an *in utero* diagnosis; they mentioned continuation of pregnancy in only 37% of these cases. Likewise, in a survey of more than 700 obstetricians, Heuser, Eller, and Byrne (2012) observe that "Nearly 100% of respondents discuss pregnancy termination for both uniformly and commonly lethal anomalies" (392). Although they do not explicitly define these terms in their study, they point to anencephaly and bilateral renal agenesis as instances of uniformly lethal conditions; they list trisomy 13, trisomy 18, and alobar holoprosencephaly as examples of severe commonly lethal conditions. In the same survey, only 11% would support or encourage a parent who requests support measures to ensure a live birth. In the case of uniformly lethal anomalies, nearly 30% of physicians would refuse to comply with this request; in the case of severe commonly lethal anomalies, 18% would refuse such of request. Nearly 73% of obstetricians would actively discourage such a choice in the case of uniformly lethal anomalies and 66% would actively discourage this choice in the case of severe commonly lethal anomalies. Even in contexts where parents ask for no interventions to ensure a live birth, around 30% of physicians report that they still would not encourage such a choice.[7]

Furthermore, families report that the language physicians use to describe their child or the child's condition can convey negative attitudes about the child's life or his value. Consider, again, Guon et al.'s (2014) study in which parents were informed that

> their baby would likely die before or at the time of birth (94%),
> that their baby would not live for more than a few months (88%),

that the condition of their baby was lethal or incompatible with life (93%), that their child would be a vegetable (55%), that their baby would destroy their family or their marriage (28%), and that if their baby survived, he would live a meaningless life (55%) or a life of suffering (68%).

(312)

Given the available evidence, only some of this language is warranted. It is highly probable that a child diagnosed with trisomy 13 or 18 will die before or shortly after birth. Nonetheless, a failure to indicate that there are children who defy these odds can suggest that this is not a real possibility for the family. The terms 'lethal' or 'fatal' should be used only with significant qualifications. These terms can be employed in clinically appropriate ways: significantly life-limiting conditions increase the likelihood of a quick death.[8] But there are children who survive beyond expectations and active interventions can sometimes increase longevity.

As the preceding quote indicates, medically accurate language is often coupled with terms that appear critical of their choice to continue the pregnancy.[9] The phrases and terms such as 'incompatible with life,' 'vegetable,' 'meaningless life,' 'life of suffering,' along with the claim that the child's survival will destroy the family or marriage are neither clinically accurate nor morally neutral.

Lathrop and VandeVusse (2011) report that mothers whose children were diagnosed *in utero* with a significantly life-limiting condition felt invalidated by language that seemed to devalue their unborn children or their identity as mothers.[10] To claim that the unborn child's life is "incompatible with life" may signal that the clinician does not value the child. Language of this sort is particularly painful when it was uttered by physicians because of their "special authority in the health care setting" (260). One mother stated,

> Well, the doctor said we have to terminate: 'It's non-compatible with life.' . . . who are they to say that? You know what I mean? Who are they to take all this wonderful, beautiful experience that we had away just because they feel it's non-compatible with life?
>
> (260)

It is important to note that this use of language may not be rooted in vicious motives. Wilkinson et al. (2012, 1304–5) offer several possible explanations for the use of the language of 'lethal' or 'fatal' conditions in the context of adverse *in utero* diagnoses. They note that some physicians may be unaware of new evidence of longevity for particular conditions. Others may be uncomfortable with prognostic uncertainty and, as a result, look for ways to help to ease the discomfort both they and the families have in making timely decisions. Some may judge that families may experience less discomfort with the thought of terminating the pregnancy (or in pursuing palliative care) if they think of the condition is lethal. Some may be seeking to ease burdens on other healthcare providers who would be charged with providing care in difficult circumstances. In some cases, it seems that their words and actions may be motivated by moral concerns to restore a family's sense of control or to alleviate their suffering. If this is true with respect to terms like 'lethal' that admit of a qualified clinical meaning, one may argue that similar motives may move physicians to use other value-laden terms like 'incompatible with life.'

Framing the family's choices with language that is either inapt or value-laden, however, can convey the message that families are not welcome within institutional spaces of medical care.[11] Even if there are admirable motivations underlying this use of language, physicians and genetic counselors can contribute to an unwelcoming ethos. This is compounded by what families can learn by seeking out alternative sources of information. Wilkinson, Crespigny, and Xafis (2014) observe that

> the Internet has provided families with the ability to do their own research and encounter alternate perspectives on their child's condition. Within seconds of searching for 'trisomy 18' a parent may see pictures of many older children with trisomy 18, smiling and happy, strong evidence against 'incompatibility with life'.
>
> (307)

If physicians describe conditions such as trisomy 18 in ways that contradict these personal narratives, affected families may suspect that the point of using such language is to ensure a particular outcome—the termination of the pregnancy. Parents may lack sufficient evidence to justify this characterization of healthcare providers' motives or intent, but the discrepancy between a physician's words and these narratives can signal to the family that healthcare providers do not want to care for them.

At the same time, it is not clear that the availability of these programs is sufficient to ensure that families can access available care. In a recent study, Marc-Aurele et al. (2017) examined referrals to an established perinatal hospice program over a six-year period of time from one high-risk fetal diagnostic center in San Diego County, California. Of the 332 cases, around 40% of the affected families chose expectant management of the pregnancy. Only thirty-six women in total were referred for perinatal palliative consultations following an adverse diagnosis and, of these women, only twenty-six received palliative care.[12] Less than half of the women who could have benefitted from perinatal hospice consultation received the opportunity. At the same time, 56% of the affected families chose to receive "therapeutic abortion" (179). Marc-Aurele et al. (2017) observe that the legal restrictions governing abortion combined with the average gestational age at time of confirmed diagnosis create a context in which "the chance to provide a palliative care consult before women elect to undergo therapeutic abortion is within only a few days" (182). During the time of this study, the average time between diagnosis and referral for palliative care was approximately seven weeks.

There are social structures external to medical institutions that can reinforce the family's sense that their child and, by extension, the family itself is not welcome within spaces of medical care. Consider, for instance, the routine practice of prenatal screening. Ultrasound screenings and other noninvasive tests are a common part of obstetrical care. But these scans have, as a central aim, the discovery of markers for disease or disability. Knowledge of this sort can be helpful: families and physicians are better able to anticipate needs that can be addressed at birth. But the knowledge they provide forces individuals to choose how they will address potentially negative findings. Will they welcome a child who has a condition that will mean death or certain disability? Given the rarity of many of these conditions, it is unlikely that most families will have to ask this question of themselves. But the widespread use of screening technology ensures that many will be forced to make a choice on the basis of the information gleaned from these scans. Sarah Williams (2018) notes:

> As a practice, prenatal scanning both teaches and reinforces particular ways of thinking about the human person. It teaches the pregnant couple to ask: Is this child physically normal? The question is asked as if it were of primary importance. Whether or not the scan results reveal fetal abnormality, the practice makes everyone ask this question at a relatively early stage of pregnancy. It may only be a tiny statistical minority of parents who choose with much grief and heartache to terminate a pregnancy because of fetal abnormality (and such parents should never be judged). But the fact that we have an almost universal social practice that renders acceptable the *idea* of terminating the life of a child whose physical capacities are suboptimal affects every one of us. This idea is further reinforced by a legal structure that makes such an idea not only *plausible* but also *permissible* and *possible* right up to full term. Moreover, we have sophisticated language to cloak the idea in moral neutrality, and we have a definition of "quality of life" to explain why such an idea is right and necessary.
>
> (153–4)

I cannot address this particular social structure at length in this present context, but it is worth noting that routine screening for genetic conditions and disability when it is accompanied by overt or subtle pressures to terminate a pregnancy is a social structure that can narrow a family's options without their awareness. If termination is typical in these contexts, failing to comply with this norm may invite criticism from medical professionals who judge that the parents are choosing unwisely.[13]

The evidence surveyed in this section offers a portrait of unwelcoming attitudes, practices, and social structures families may experience following an adverse *in utero* diagnosis. Active resistance to an affected family's choice to continue the pregnancy or a lack of institutional support for their choices can leave a family on the threshold of care, experiencing the diminishing effects of an unmet need for welcome. Professional communities and institutions can offer a better way—a structured program of care that addresses the family's need to be welcomed into a space of protection and care. This need is a focal concern of the virtue of hospitality.

III. Hospitality as an Individual Virtue

The term 'hospitality' admits of a wide range of uses. I do not seek to question varied uses of the term 'hospitality' or contest alternative analyses of hospitality; instead, my aim in this section is to offer a profile that can plausibly be construed as a virtue. Traditionally, hospitality has been identified with the activity of welcoming and providing for strangers who are in need. The term 'strangers' refers broadly to those who are vulnerable because they are outside of the protective structures of communal life. The stranger's social exclusion means that he lacks both the resources to care for vital needs and the standing to make claims on the resources of a particular community. Extending hospitality is an opening of communal boundaries and resources to tend to the needs of the stranger. But an analysis of the virtue of hospitality must do more than describe its behavioral expression.[14] It is, in part, a disposition to fulfill tasks appropriate to the social role of a *host*, but it is also a virtue that manifests in distinct patterns of affective, motivational, behavioral, and cognitive response.

The hospitable person displays a heightened sensitivity and attentiveness to the needs of those who are vulnerable because of their estrangement. He is moved by these needs: they present themselves as a task to which he is called to address. In part, this is because hospitality transforms how one perceives or construes the stranger in need. He is not an object of pitiable concern; rather, he is a vulnerable individual deserving care. He is not a mere stranger; he is a potential guest worthy of invitation, welcome regard, care, and fellowship. In receiving and properly acknowledging the guest, the hospitable person recognizes the guest's deep need and value.

The hospitable person opens himself to a relationship of mutuality and reciprocity. Hospitality is not mere charity or generosity; it is an invitation to share a common space together (even if it is for a short duration).[15] The hospitable person is disinclined to erect or maintain impermeable boundaries between himself and those on the outside. He willingly and gladly opens himself and his community to care for the guest's needs. And the receptivity characteristic of this virtue enables the host to appreciate the gift he receives in welcoming the guest. He is engaged in an encounter of both giving to and receiving from a person who is no longer estranged because he has become a welcomed and honored guest. But the hospitable person's motivation is not self-serving; he is motivated by an other-regarding concern for the guest's needs.

It is instructive to contrast the virtue of hospitality with several vices. But one should first note that are multiple ways in which one may fail to possess or to exercise the virtue of hospitality without being an inhospitable person. For instance, a person who feels moved by the needs of the stranger, is motivated to respond to his need, recognizes his value and inherent dignity, and invites him into a space of care may still fail to display the virtue of hospitality if he fails to open himself to a relationship of mutual regard and receptive concern. This person is not vicious even if he fails to express the virtue of hospitality in its fullness. A failure in one dimension of hospitality does not entail that one has an opposing vice; it merely indicates that one does not yet possess the virtue of hospitality fully or completely.

The vices of inhospitality, however, are not immature or incomplete expressions of hospitality. They are patterned forms of entrenched or habitual inhospitality with their own distinct dispositional signatures.[16] In what follows, I begin by providing profiles of two vices of inhospitality: *hostility* and *indifference*.[17] I also profile a counterfeit form of welcome that is rooted in a dispositional *partiality* for specific types of privileged guests. The selectivity characteristic of dispositional *partiality* reflects a skewed understanding of the concerns at the heart of hospitality.

At the most extreme, a person may be characterized by a dispositional *hostility* toward those who are vulnerable. The *hostile* person is moved by a kind of antipathy or enmity toward the stranger. There are a number of distinct concerns that might feed such hostility, including a basic hatred for or fear of those outside one's intimate circle. Regardless of the motivations, hostility always expresses itself in a willingness to reject the stranger because he is a stranger. The vice of hostility disposes a person to a heightened sensitivity toward the presence of strangers on the boundaries of his space. But he fails to see them as worthy recipients of protection and care and he feels no sense of responsibility to tend to their needs. Instead, he is disposed to prevent the stranger from coming near; he barricades his community from any kind of encroachment on their space. He refuses to invite the stranger in; he will not share space with him; and he is inclined to push him away. Hostility expresses itself in a willingness to exercise violence against the stranger. The stranger is not a potential guest; he is a likely enemy.

Hostility is not the only form of vicious inhospitality. A person can be characteristically unwelcoming without being hostile; he may display an entrenched indifference or unconcern for strangers. The indifferent person consistently fails to perceive or to be moved by the needs of the stranger. The stranger's vulnerability simply fails to register, or if it does, it fails to register as salient or worthy of attention. If he is confronted by these needs, the indifferent person fails to respond with welcome regard because he has a settled habit of being unmoved by the need for welcome. Dispositional indifference dampens any natural, or reflexive, twinge of concern that may give rise to the sense that he is called to address their need. He can entertain the thought that it would be good for someone else to respond, but he fails to see any reason why he should be the one to act on the stranger's behalf. As a result, he fails to invite the person in; he will not seek his good and will not enact a relationship characterized by mutuality and reciprocity.

Some forms of indifference are bare expressions of dispositional insensitivity or inattentiveness. But, at times, indifference is motivated by a commitment to other personal projects. To borrow a metaphor, these projects act as a centripetal force, drawing all of one's attention and care away from the stranger and his needs.[18] Indifference of this sort displays itself in a closed-off stance toward the stranger. Indifference to the stranger's needs insulates one from the felt need to receive them into a space of care. Hospitality, by contrast, acts as a kind of centrifugal force, drawing one toward those on the periphery.

There are other dispositions that fail to manifest the excellence expressed in the exercise of hospitality because they display themselves in counterfeit forms of welcome. One common form is a disposition to welcome only those whose prominence would confer some important benefit on the host. In this case, the motivation for inviting and welcoming the other is the advantage conferred upon the host in receiving a person of importance. This self-serving motivation is incompatible with the virtuous expression of hospitable welcome. Another common form involves a disposition to offer provision for needs but only if or when the stranger makes an explicit request for care. A person with this disposition fails to appreciate that the socially disadvantaged are unlikely to request care, especially if they perceive potential hosts as uninviting. This disposition exhibits a circumscribed sensitivity to the concerns at the heart of hospitality.

Although I have distinguished between hospitality and both its opposing vices and counterfeit expressions, one may have a clearer sense for the nature of the virtue of hospitality by distinguishing it further from other aligned virtues. As I noted in Chapter 1, hospitality is one virtue within an allocentric cluster of traits that are rooted in a concern for the wellbeing of others. Although these virtues are interconnected, they can be distinguished by attending to the distinct needs that elicit these virtues and their characteristic behavioral, affective, and social expressions. Here, it is worth dwelling briefly on some of the distinctive dimensions of hospitality in relation to those virtues I describe more fully in subsequent chapters. This discussion will be deepened in later chapters when we have full portraits of these aligned traits in view. Although there are differences, it is important to bear in mind that specific types of vulnerability often co-occur and, thus, virtuous responses to need often require the simultaneous expression of allied virtues.

Hospitality differs from allocentric hope, solidarity, and compassion in its focus on the vulnerabilities occasioned by social exclusion or estrangement. Allocentric hope focuses on needs resulting from another person's near despair in conditions where there are goods available and worthy of pursuit. Although social alienation may be a cause of one's loss of hope, one can resign oneself to hopelessness or despair even if one is a full-fledged member of a community. Solidarity focuses on the needs occasioned by isolation. Although social exclusion is a kind of isolation, one can experience isolation or solitude even if one has full standing within a community. Being a full-fledged member of a community is not sufficient to experience the kind of union characteristic of solidary relations. Compassion focuses on the needs of those who are suffering and involves a characteristic willingness to share in another's suffering—that is, to take it on as a shared project. Although alienation or estrangement often is a source of suffering, one can be a stranger to a community without suffering because of one's social exclusion. The focal concern of hospitality is the needs of the stranger, but this alienation is not necessarily a cause of suffering. Compassion takes a more general focus in its concern for both strangers and intimates.

Given this focus on the needs of those who are estranged from communal spaces, the hospitable person is much more sensitive to those on the periphery and who are potentially alienated. For the hospitable person, what is most salient in a situation of recognized need is the fact that the person is a stranger whom he could host as a guest. His sensitivity to a person's alienation creates in him a strong desire to invite the person into a space where he can experience belonging and care. He may be concerned about the person's perceived hopelessness, isolation, or suffering, but this is a consequence of his realization that social estrangement can cause despair, isolation, and suffering. The sensitivities of the person expressing allocentric hope are directed toward a person who is near despair and unable to see available goods that are worthy of his anticipation and pursuit. Likewise, the attention of the person with the virtue of solidarity focuses in a distinct direction. He is sensitive to the isolation people may be experiencing regardless of whether they are within or outside the community. And the compassionate person is sensitive to suffering independent of these considerations of communal membership. None of these virtues is specifically attuned to the individual's place or social standing as outside the community.

Finally, one can distinguish these virtues by attending to their characteristic expression. Hospitality expresses itself chiefly in its welcome of those who are alienated into a space of belonging while allocentric hope characteristically expresses itself in its communication of a vision of the goods that are possible and worthy of another's hopeful pursuit. Both hospitality and solidarity emphasize union with those in need, but there is difference in the direction of their characteristic movements. Hospitality typically expresses itself in an invitation to a stranger into a space of belonging, protection, and care while solidarity typically issues in a movement outward to join with those experiencing hardship. Like hospitality, compassion often expresses itself in care for the one who is suffering, but its focus is on alleviating or helping the individual to endure the suffering. Hospitality, on the other hand, focuses primarily on addressing the need for social standing. A lack of social standing may not, by itself, be a source of suffering. It creates significant vulnerability—a need that can elicit moral concern. But this vulnerability may not be a source of suffering. Thus, it may not elicit compassion. This discussion is too brief, but I return to questions about the individuation of these virtues again in the chapters that follow.

At this point, one might have a sense for the basic contours of the virtue of hospitality. Hospitality is a virtue that takes the need for welcome as a focal object of concern. In contexts where individuals or groups fall outside the protection of the community or in times when individuals or groups are alienated or estranged, their need for welcome care and regard triggers a cascade of affective, behavioral, cognitive, and relational responses that address this need. The hospitable person feels moved by the needs of the stranger and desires to address his needs. He invites the stranger into a space of care in order to provide for his needs. He sees the stranger as one worthy of relationship and care. He takes the stranger's need as a reason to enact a relational bond with him as a guest. Even when these bonds are temporary (because the needs for care or protection are no longer present), they connect host and guest together in a relationship of mutuality and reciprocity. On the account I am developing, however, virtues are excellences crucial to the flourishing of individuals within community. One may recognize hospitality as a human excellence but wonder whether such a trait is crucial to living a fulfilling human life. So, in order to complete this profile, I need to articulate a sense of the value of hospitality. Although I cannot offer a full defense in the space of this chapter, I can point to some important considerations that could ground such an account.

First, one ought to consider the ways the virtue of hospitality benefits the stranger and potential guest. The most obvious benefit he receives is the protection of a community willing to tend to his vulnerability and need. The care and belonging he receives can address the diminishing effects of his social exclusion. He also receives the gift of an enacted bond of concern with those who see him as deserving of care. By themselves, these bonds are a source of comfort for one whose exclusion has left him without the opportunities for mutuality and reciprocity in relationship. But more than this, the invitation into a space of care is an invitation into a space where one is recognized and respected as an individual with value. Given the lack of standing strangers experience, the exercise of hospitality elevates the recipient by acknowledging his value. Beyond these immediate benefits to a particular stranger, the virtue of hospitality has a more general benefit to strangers considered as a group. The exercise of hospitality challenges the fixity of boundaries between those within and those outside the community. Hospitality can dissolve arbitrary and artificial divisions that typically separate people within social groups. For this reason, the exercise of hospitable welcome can eradicate barriers to care and protection that systematically harm those who are most vulnerable.

Second, one should consider the wide range of benefits hospitality confers upon its possessor. Individuals with a hospitable disposition possess a deepened understanding of the locus of individual dignity. The value of a person is something inherent; it is not reducible to membership within a particular social group. Thus, hospitality frees one to consider the true source and value of individual life. Consequently, it makes the hospitable person sensitive to the expansive nature of moral concern; the needs of those beyond his own community should elicit his caring concern. Failing to attend to the needs of a person on the margins of one's community simply because he is not an intimate is an expression of deficient regard for one in need. The hospitable person is sensitive to the ways virtue calls him to act on the stranger's behalf.

Additionally, this kind of *other-regarding* focus is an expression of an important human excellence. It is a posture of committed care for the person in need that reflects a commitment to the good. It orients one toward the goal of addressing the stranger's vulnerability with fitting care. In this way, one displays a posture of *being for* the good of the stranger. It also orients the host to the person as a guest. This kind of allocentric regard is, by itself, expressive of a good in human life—the good of *being for* others. Robert Adams (2006) contends that this kind of orientation enables one to

> live in a larger and richer universe of relations. In giving oneself unreservedly to other persons or to larger goods one escapes from isolation. One moves with freedom, and probably with much richer perceptiveness, in a space of values in which one's life can have significance in relation to those other persons and goods and not merely in relation to oneself.
>
> (2006, 77)

Hospitality is also a helpful aid to the development of good communities. Given that we are all fragile and dependent beings, we all are susceptible to the kinds of social exclusion or alienation characteristic of those who are strangers. We are all potentially in need of the care, protection, and provision of others who welcome us into their communities. Thus, fostering individual hospitality is crucial to cultivating social conditions integral to addressing both the vulnerability of others and one's own vulnerability. This point provides reason to think of the virtue of hospitality as a virtue of acknowledged dependence. As MacIntyre (1999a) notes, we need virtues of uncalculated giving and receiving that open us to the needs of those outside our intimate bonds. Familial and friendship bonds may ground care for those with profound needs, but we need virtues that move us to care for those who do not currently belong to our communities. Virtues of acknowledged dependence move individuals to extend care simply because the other is in need. This care seeks to address the need fully and without demanding a reciprocal exchange. Hospitable welcome is fitting because the stranger is one in need and deserving of care because of his value. Given that virtues of acknowledged dependence are virtues crucial for human fulfillment, a failure to cultivate and practice hospitality within our communities is a failure to foster a culture in which individuals are likely to flourish.

I have offered an extended profile of hospitality as an individual disposition. But the central aim of this chapter is to argue that perinatal hospice is a common project that manifests hospitable welcome. Therefore, I need to augment this sketch to show how particular professional communities and their social structures can manifest the virtue of hospitality.

IV. Hospitality, Common Projects, and Facilitating Social Structures

I maintain that a hospitable professional community or institution is one that devotes itself to a common project of hospitable welcome. Participation in this common project involves attentiveness and sensitivity to the needs of strangers, a characteristic care or concern to address vulnerabilities rooted in the stranger's lack of standing, and coordinated activities aimed at addressing these needs.

Participating in a common project of this sort is more than the commitment to a shared endeavor; it involves a particular type of care for the family as a fundamental feature of a collective pursuit. A group that cares properly for the common project of hospitable welcome is engaged in an endeavor to welcome the guest in a manner that is sensitive to his vulnerabilities and needs. Furthermore, they do so because they appreciate and value the persons whom they receive into their care. It is unlikely that a professional community or institution will engage in a common project of hospitable welcome if few of its members care properly for the goals and concerns of the project. Participation in this common project involves an orientation of *being for* those who find themselves estranged or alienated from spaces of belonging and care. This kind of other-regarding concern by itself requires a commitment to open the community to those who have not yet been received into a space of care. Devotion to the aims of this common project is an important motivational component of reliably fulfilling a role within the joint pursuit. Individual members of a community contribute to this collective endeavor by fulfilling a role within an integrated or coordinated effort.[19]

We might contrast this with a community or institution that fails to display the kinds of attentiveness, concern, and collective engagement in welcoming those who are vulnerable and in need. Some communities or institutions fail to display this kind of concern because they are hostile toward the stranger. Other communities or institutions may not be hostile, but they display entrenched forms of collective inattentiveness, unconcern, and indifference. Moreover, communities and institutions may display counterfeit expression of partial welcome. A community or institution may fail to engage in this kind of common project even if many of the members within the community or institution are individually welcoming. Strangers may experience welcome regard, care, and protection from individuals within the community without experiencing this from the community or institution as a whole. The collective failure to exercise the virtue of hospitality, however, is not equivalent to possessing or manifesting vices of inhospitality.

More should be said about social structures and their contributions to a common project of hospitable welcome. As I noted previously, social structures act to frame the types of interactions and encounters one experiences within a particular context.[20] Both internal and external social structures shape institutions and their character. Some internal structures are explicitly encoded in protocols, policies, and procedures that define and delimit the nature of expected practice. Other internal structures are implicit, a part of the culture of the institution, often emerging dynamically over time or through the influence of important members within the institution. External social structures—such as explicit economic incentives and legal norms or social norms and assumptions implicit in the broader culture—can frame an institution's characteristic activities. These external structures can shape common expectations about the nature, scope, and limits of an institution's typical practice.

Some types of social structure enable individuals to act and express hospitality more readily while other structures may make the expression of hospitality much more difficult. We might characterize hospitable social structures as facilitating structures—that is, social structures that enable individuals, communities, and institutions to engage in a common project of hospitable welcome more readily and with greater consistency. An inhospitable social structure, by contrast, would be one that either inhibits engagement in such a project or facilitates commitment to projects that express either the vices of hostility or indifference or the counterfeit expressions of partial welcome.

Up to this point, much of this discussion has been at a theoretical level. It is important, however, to show how one may apply this analysis to the concrete experience of families who have received an adverse *in utero* diagnosis. A concrete portrait of hospitality expressed by professional communities and medical institutions should begin by identifying the relevant actors and the distinct roles they play in this context. In particular, it is important to identify those who are strangers (and potential guests) and those who are potential hosts. I noted earlier that the hospitable person is disposed to perceive strangers as individuals with inherent worth and value. Within the context of life-limiting diagnoses, there are two potential subjects of hospitable concern: the unborn child and families. One may wonder whether the construal of an unborn child as a subject of hospitable concern requires a commitment to the view that the unborn child has moral status. If it does, it is not clear that the *virtue-based* defense I am offering is independent of the *moral status* defense outlined in Chapter 1. There I noted that the defense I am developing could be construed as a supplement to extant defenses. If the analysis I have offered in this chapter is apt, then one could augment a *moral status* defense by adopting this *virtue-based* analysis of hospitable concern for the unborn child. Endorsement of the moral status of the unborn child would give one reason to treat him as a subject of hospitable concern.

Although one could develop such a defense, it is not clear that the analysis I have offered requires commitment to the view that the unborn child has moral status. One may treat an unborn child as a potential subject of hospitable concern even if one is not prepared to endorse the view that the unborn child has full moral status. Consider, for instance, the clinician who treats the unborn child *as if* he has moral status because he refuses to foreclose on this possibility. This stance does not require endorsement of a controversial metaphysical view of personhood. Or, consider the clinician who treats the unborn child as a potential subject of hospitable concern because the child's family construes the child as an individual with inherent worth and value. In this context, failure to treat the unborn child as an individual with worth significantly compromises one's ability to welcome the family into the space of care. So, one can treat the unborn child *as if* he has moral status so that one can properly welcome the family. Treating the unborn child *as if* he has moral status is, thus, a means of welcoming individuals one sees as potential guests. It is proper to the role of the host to welcome them in this way. These responses are an initial attempt to address the concern that my *virtue-based* defense depends upon the moral status of the unborn child, but more will need to be said concerning the connections between my defense and other extant analyses. I return to this discussion with greater depth in Chapter 7.

For the purposes of the analysis in this chapter, I focus instead on the affected family as strangers and subjects of hospitable concern. To identify these families as strangers is, in part, to indicate that they are vulnerable because their circumstances are potentially alienating. Their experiences are relatively rare; unlike most families who experience typical pregnancies, these families are susceptible to being left outside the space of a welcoming environment of care. Given that the choice to continue a pregnancy is atypical, physicians, genetic counselors, nurses, medical institutions, and even the family's personal community may not expect families to continue the pregnancy.[21] They may be uninviting and unprepared to welcome the family because they assumed the family would comply with the standard expectations.

If the family occupies the role of stranger, hospitable professional communities and institutions are those who enact the role of host. They take the family into their ambit of concern and seek to address their physical, psychological, emotional, and spiritual needs as they anticipate the child's birth and death. Offering a hospitable environment begins with the physician's diagnosis of a life-limiting condition. Physicians and specialists ensure that they carefully describe all of the available options for the family. By describing alternatives such as perinatal hospice and how they may access such care, physicians have already invited them into a space of care.

In addition to this, hospitable professional communities and institutional structures will be careful to avoid framing a family's choice in ways that are unwelcoming. In delivering a diagnosis, a hospitable community will seek to provide adequate space or time to consider the various options. Healthcare providers will employ language that is medically accurate and sensitive to prognostic uncertainties. Physicians can acknowledge the severe nature of these conditions without expressing language that skews a family's vision of the goods they may realize through the choice to continue the pregnancy. Uses of terms such as 'fatal,' 'lethal,' or 'incompatible with life,' can be deeply problematic in these contexts.[22] As I noted earlier, a charitable understanding of the use of these terms is that they are intended to convey the seriousness of the conditions. These conditions cannot be cured and they substantially increase the likelihood of death either before or shortly after birth. Physicians may intend these terms to be neutral, but they can convey a sense that the child's life is not worth living. Families may construe this language as suggesting that the child's life is meaningless.

If the family chooses to continue an affected pregnancy, professional communities and institutions can express hospitable welcome in additional ways. First, they can help the family to develop a plan of care for the remainder of the pregnancy and after delivery.[23] They can help families prepare for birth, death, or even the remote possibility of ongoing life. They can seek to create a network of support for the family by connecting the family with therapists and social workers to address psychosocial needs. They can coordinate with the delivery site to ensure that there is clear communication and a working plan for delivery. As the delivery date approaches, neonatologists can work with parents to shape a plan of palliative care following birth to ensure that the child does not experience unnecessary pain. They can construct contingency plans for more aggressive treatment if that is warranted. They can also connect families with organizations, like the professional photographers associated with *Now I Lay Me Down To Sleep*, who volunteer to take pictures of the family prior to birth and after delivery in order to facilitate memory-making and to ensure that the family has meaningful keepsake photographs. Finally, they can address the family's needs following the death of the child, preemptively tending to the particular needs and questions that may occur in this context. In developing these plans, organizing the support, and communicating the family's goals and desires, professional communities attend to their need for hospitable welcome.

I can illustrate this account best by considering an exemplary case. Cole et al. (2017) describe the experiences of a family referred to the Perinatal Palliative Care and Bereavement Program at The Children's Hospital of Philadelphia following an antenatal diagnosis of trisomy 13. Trisomy 13, or Patau Syndrome, is a rare chromosomal condition in which the child inherits an extra copy of the thirteenth chromosome. Prognoses for children with trisomy 13 are typically poor. There are a range of associated anomalies including severe heart and brain defects that can leave the child extremely fragile. For children born with this condition, an overwhelming majority will die before the end of their first year of life. In a population-based study, Rasmussen et al. (2003) report that "median survival time for infants with trisomy 13 was 7 days using [Metropolitan Atlanta Congenital Defects Program] data, and the median age at death was 10 days using [Multiple-Cause Mortality Files] data" (782). They also report that "91% of infants with trisomy 13 or with trisomy 18 died within the first year of life" (782).[24]

Cole et al. (2017) note that the family's initial perinatal palliative and hospice care consultation involved discussion of the range of therapeutic modalities available to them in the event that the child was born alive. They also discussed the prognostic uncertainty concerning the child's care—factors that affect the longevity of life that they would not be able to assess until birth. This initial visit resulted in a provisional plan of care for after delivery. And this plan of care was immediately included in the mother's medical record as a guide for all subsequent visits.

After the initial consultation, a clinical psychologist met with the family to discuss psychosocial care for their four-year-old son, developing a plan for how best to prepare him for his sister's birth and death. This discussion led to a referral to a child life specialist who was able to help the family cultivate developmentally appropriate forms of language to discuss his sister's condition. They also discussed how he could be included in the process of memory-making so that he could process difficult emotions and his grief. The family was invited to bring their son with them to prenatal visits. On those occasions where they brought him, he was able to develop a relationship with a clinical psychologist and become sensitized to the hospital environment.

Throughout this process, an advanced practice registered nurse coordinated the family's care. At each appointment, she reviewed their provisional plan and gave the family opportunities to discuss their ongoing needs. She sought to confirm the details of their plan, updating it in light of new desires or goals. These meetings provided opportunities for caregivers to develop a deep understanding of the family's values, needs, and desires—an understanding that fostered a sensitive attunement to the family for the duration of their care.

Nearly thirty-six weeks into the pregnancy, the child suffered *in utero* demise and was delivered by elective cesarean section. Healthcare providers followed their plan for bonding and memory-making after birth, including "taking photos, making hand and foot molds, and eventually introducing their son to his sister" (Cole et al. 2017, 909). In the presence of the child life specialist, they sought to provide comfort and care for their son. Cole et al. (2017) write,

> After explaining that she died, the couple gave their son the choice to meet his sister and to be involved in the memory-making process. He spent his time in the post-partum recovery room shifting between getting to know his sister, playing with toys, and openly expressing his emotions to describe his current experience.
>
> (909)

Those members of the perinatal palliative care team involved in psychosocial support helped the family to follow their plan of care for the three days they were in the hospital. The family had minimal interruptions from hospital staff, allowing them time and space for "family bonding, honest grieving, and intimacy that minimized traumatic stress and aided in the beginning stages of integrating the loss into their family narrative" (Cole et al. 2017, 909). The family engaged in care-giving tasks such as bathing, dressing, and holding the child. And a clinical psychologist met with them to support them in their grief and to help prepare them to leave the hospital and return to their communities.

This case illustrates how the provision and promotion of perinatal hospice can manifest a welcoming social ethos—one in which families experience care adequate to address their potential alienation and estrangement. To employ the language from an earlier section of this chapter, this family was received into a space of care as vulnerable and honored guests. They experienced the inviting and welcoming presence of physicians, nurses, social workers, and grief counselors within an ethos of institutional support.

There is a clear difference between this kind of ethos and the unwelcoming structures and dynamics outlined at the outset of this chapter.

Addressing unwelcoming attitudes, practices, and social structures may require significant reform. In the conclusion, I consider the kinds of communal, institutional, and structural remedies crucial to ensuring that families do not experience an unmet need for welcome. I offer concrete proposals for changes that can encourage healthcare providers and medical institutions to engage well in a common project of hospitable welcome.

V. Conclusion—Fostering a Hospitable Institutional Culture

I began the chapter by highlighting the experience of a family whose choice to continue a pregnancy was met with apparent hostility. Individual healthcare providers critically questioned the value of the family's choice; the family had to fight against institutional structures that made accessing quality care arduous. In Section II, I surveyed some of the available evidence indicating that professional communities, institutions, and social structures often close themselves off from families who are open to continuing a pregnancy. The failure to engage in a common project of hospitable welcome can add to the burdens families experience in these difficult circumstances. When one contrasts these deficient forms of welcome with the hospitable welcome received within a structured perinatal hospice program, one can see why the development of these programs is crucial to addressing the needs of families who have received an adverse *in utero* diagnosis.

Given the deficiencies of many current structures, what needs to occur to foster a more hospitable welcome for families in need of care? The first step involves reforms in typical patterns of delivering significantly life-limiting diagnoses. In order to foster a hospitable institutional culture, professional communities and institutions must seek to curb those practices, policies, or protocols that display overt hostility or indifference. Altering these institutional practices may be difficult because of the ways they are deeply entrenched and encultured within medical systems. Furthermore, as I noted in Section II, they may be supported by external social structures, attitudes, and commitments that are difficult to dislodge. So, how can one address these kinds of pressures effectively?

One may not be able to change the commitments and attitudes that give rise to individual expressions of inhospitality. But professional communities and institutions can develop modes of responding that structure how individuals deliver diagnoses such that they do not unwittingly engage in practices that manifest inhospitality in its various forms. One form this may take is the practice of nondirective counseling.[25] This practice is ordered toward the elimination of pressures placed upon the family. The goal is to provide information sufficient for families to make choices consonant with their values without biasing them in one way or another.

But there is evidence that physicians and genetic counselors are strongly inclined to engage in directive counseling in cases involving antenatal diagnoses of significantly life-limiting conditions. They often direct families toward termination. So, even if the professional community has adopted nondirective counseling as the appropriate norm, it will have its intended effect only if there is a much greater commitment on the part of the healthcare providers and institutions to its consistent implementation.

Such a commitment does not guarantee that professional communities and institutions will refrain from practices that subtly pressure families to choose to terminate the pregnancy. The use of inapt and value-laden language, appeals to normalcy, expressed urgency in soliciting a decision, insensitivity to or intentional refusal to attend to prognostic uncertainty, and failure to discuss or consider serious alternatives to termination can preempt a family's full consideration of the available options. These kinds of framing effects are often rooted in attitudes and judgments that are persistent, implicit, and enculturated. It is not clear that adopting the norm of nondirective counseling as a practice will address these kinds of framing effects.

Furthermore, it is not clear that the procedural neutrality of nondirective counseling is an expression of hospitable welcome. At most, it is a structural means of alleviating overt expressions of inhospitality toward the family. Encoded within this policy is a posture of noncommitment that displays a willingness to extend welcome care only if the family chooses to continue the pregnancy. The family can interpret this neutrality as inviting only in the most qualified sense. In fact, this kind of neutrality may be akin to the counterfeit form of welcome I described previously in which one is received into a supportive environment only when one asks for care.[26] I noted that this kind of conditional welcome reflects an inadequate appreciation of the concerns at the heart of hospitality. Hospitality is more than providing care; it is a posture that disposes individuals and communities to invite those in need of welcome into a space where they can receive care. Furthermore, for families who desire the opportunity to care for their child, the neutrality of nondirective counseling may seem like an expression of utter indifference.[27]

So, fostering a more hospitable culture requires reform in the common practices of delivering adverse *in utero* diagnoses. Adopting a policy of nondirective counseling may be a first step toward promoting institutional change, but, by itself, it is not a manifestation of hospitable welcome. One must do more than insist on nondirective counseling to ensure that families experience a hospitable welcome within institutions devoted to their care. Fostering a more hospitable culture begins by increasing the awareness of and the accessibility to perinatal hospice. Physicians and counselors can discuss with families what kind of care is available even if there are no structured programs within their immediate vicinity. Exemplar programs such as the one discussed earlier provide a map for how one may develop and provide such care. But more than promotion, fostering a hospitable institutional culture for families in need of welcome should involve the creation of structured programs of care. Better organized programs in perinatal hospice are much easier to discuss with families. They offer greater welcome because there are institutional supports built directly into the delivery of care. Families would not need to create a plan of care out of nothing. There would be healthcare providers present and available to them to help fashion and coordinate care, connecting them with a team of professionals who can support them for the duration of the pregnancy. The promotion and provision of perinatal hospice programs is a way of creating and extending a welcoming ethos of care. A commitment to this common project is a manifestation of the virtue of hospitality.

Notes

1 See Reist (2006) for a catalog of narratives of this sort.
2 For evidence challenging these assertions, see Janvier, Farlow, and Wilfond (2012) and Guon et al. (2014).
3 See Berg, Paulsen, and Carter (2013); Côté-Arsenault and Denny-Koelsch (2011); English and Hessler (2013); Farlow (2009, 2011); Farrelly et al. (2012); Guon et al. (2014); Redlinger-Grosse et al. (2002); Thiele (2010, 2011); Walker, Miller, and Dalton (2008); Wilkinson (2012); and Wilkinson et al. (2012).
4 For discussions of these kinds of pressures, see, in particular, Guon et al. (2014); Lathrop and VandeVusse (2011); and Wilkinson et al. (2012). See Yoon, Rasinski, and Curlin (2010) for broad discussions of current debates concerning directive and nondirective counseling.
5 Directive counseling of this sort is not necessarily rooted in negative attitudes or judgments about the child, the family, or their choice. Nonetheless, actively encouraging the family to terminate the pregnancy may involve implicit commitment to a number of contested views concerning the moral status of the unborn child, the nature and moral value of suffering, and the goods that can be realized through continuing a pregnancy. I address these questions more fully in Chapter 7.
6 In Breeze et al.'s (2007) study, the median time between confirmed diagnosis and the decision to terminate or continue the pregnancy was one-and-a-half days (F56).
7 For further discussion of this study, see Wilkinson et al. (2012).
8 For critical discussion of the language of 'lethal congenital malformations,' see Wilkinson, de Crespigny, and Xafis (2014).
9 Guon et al. (2014) also report that those families who sought active interventions for children were born alive reported "feeling judged" by healthcare providers for these choices (315).
10 See Lathrop and VandeVusse (2011) for further discussion of invalidating language.
11 For further discussion of potential reasons physicians employ terms such as 'lethal' or 'incompatible with life' see Wilkinson et al. (2012).
12 This is consistent with results in Leuthner and Jones (2007).
13 Families may experience unwelcoming encounters within their personal communities. For a vivid description of these interactions, see Williams's (2018, 35–37) description of the ways acquaintances among the faculty at Oxford

responded to her decision to continue a pregnancy after learning that her daughter, Cerian, had thanatophoric dysplasia, a severe skeletal defect. One colleague asked her bluntly whether her husband was forcing her to carry to term. Another colleague offered an argument that she had a moral obligation to terminate the pregnancy because Cerian's life would be suboptimal.

14 One will not always find hospitality among canonical lists of traditional virtues. But a number of distinct religious traditions have held that the failure to extend hospitality constitutes a moral failure—in particular, a failure to provide what one owes to those in need. Within the Jewish and Christian scriptures, for instance, there are explicit instructions to provide for the needs of the stranger. For discussion of hospitality in the Jewish scriptures, see Hobbs (2001). For extended discussions of Christian reflections on the virtue of hospitality, see Bretherton (2006); Newman (2007); Oden (2001); Pohl (1999); and Reynolds (2008). For a recent discussion of the import of hospitality for a project in Christian theodicy, see Timpe and Cobb (2017). For some recent philosophical reflections concerning the nature of hospitality, see Conway (2009) and Telfer (1995).

15 Traditionally, hospitality is construed as a moral response to a tangible and temporally bound need. At some point, the guest will no longer need the protection and care of the host. So, there is a boundary on the ongoing provision of hospitality. See Wrobleski (2012) for further discussion. I agree that most instances of hospitality have this kind of temporal boundary, but as a disposition, hospitality involves a reluctance to prescribe an end point of this sort. The hospitable person is disposed to remain open to providing protection and care for as long as the guest is in need. For this reason, he is not vigilantly concerned with signs that there is no longer a need.

16 It is worth emphasizing that one could fail to possess or to exercise the virtue of hospitality without being an inhospitable person. I am inclined to endorse Christian Miller's view that most people possess mixed traits—dispositions that fall somewhere between virtue and vice. This is consistent with some rare cases of individuals who are exceptionally virtuous or vicious. For defense of this view, see Miller (2013, 2014, 2017).

17 In this chapter, most of my focus is on vices of deficiency. This is, in part, because deficient forms of welcome are much more common than excessive expressions of welcome regard. Nonetheless, it is worth noting that there could be instances of habitually *excessive* welcome. There may be ways in which an undiscerning, profligate receptivity to others may undermine or defeat the real aims of hospitality. The point of hospitality is defeated if it fails to target those who are genuinely in need of care and protection because of their estrangement. These possibilities, however remote, show that the virtue of hospitality requires the exercise of prudence. See Wrobleski (2012) for further discussions of the potential limitations that flow from the prudent exercise of hospitality.

18 I borrow the metaphor from G.K. Chesterton (1936, 28), who uses it for a different purpose.

19 It is possible to participate individually in this effort without caring deeply or adequately for its goals. If a person identifies with the community or institution and its projects, or if he cares deeply for the other members of the community or the institution, or if he displays a deep commitment to fulfilling his role within a community or institution, he may be motivated to do his part in extending a hospitable welcome to the stranger even if he is not individually hospitable.

20 For further discussion on social structures, see Anderson (2012); Haslanger (2012); MacIntyre (1999b); Porpora (1989); and Smith (2010).

21 See Benute et al. (2012); Hassed et al. (1993); Lakovschek, Streubel, and Ulm (2011); Sandelowski and Barroso (2005); Sandelowski and Jones (1996); Schechtman et al. (2002); Wilkinson et al. (2012); and Wool (2011).

22 For further discussion, see Wilkinson et al. (2012).

23 For discussion, see English and Hessler (2013).

24 But they acknowledge that their study did not allow them to determine whether children who defied these odds benefitted from "aggressive care" (Rasmussen et al. 2003, 782). For further discussions of trisomy 13 and survival, see Peroos et al. (2012).

25 See Yoon, Rasinski, and Curlin (2010) contend that nondirective counseling has become a norm within certain specializations within the United States.

26 One might argue that nondirective counseling is the best one can do within the current structures because expressing the welcome regard I have described might be construed as a kind of inhospitality for families who intend to terminate the pregnancy. This is an important concern, but I cannot address it fully here. Nonetheless, it is important to note that very few families who intend to pursue this option experience medical institutions as unwelcoming. Furthermore, if the evidence I have described in this chapter is correct, an overwhelming majority of physicians and geneticists offer termination without any hesitancy. On the other hand, a significant proportion of these same groups often fail to describe the possibilities of comfort-maximizing measures at birth as an alternative. Nondirective counseling may be an improvement over open hostility or indifference, but the current practices of nondirective counseling may not be sufficient to make these alternatives a live option for families who would like to consider them.

27 I have focused here on hospitable concern for the family, but it is worth noting that if the unborn child has moral status, the neutrality of nondirective counseling is an expression of inhospitality toward the unborn child. I cannot address this concern here, but I return to it in Chapter 7.

References

Adams, Robert. 2006. *A Theory of Virtue: Excellence in Being for the Good.* Oxford: Clarendon Press.

Anderson, Elizabeth. 2012. "Epistemic Justice as a Virtue of Social Institutions." *Social Epistemology* 26 (2): 163–73.

Benute, Gláucia R.G., Roseli M.Y. Nomura, Adolfo W. Liao, Maria de Lourdes Brizot, Mara de Lucia, and M. Zugaib. 2012. "Feelings of Women Regarding End-of-life Decision Making after Ultrasound Diagnosis of a Lethal Fetal Malformation." *Midwifery* 28 (4): 472–5.

Berg, Siri F., Odd G. Paulsen, and Brian Carter. 2013. "Why Were They in Such a Hurry to See Her Die?" *American Journal of Hospice and Palliative Medicine* 30 (4): 406–8.

Breeze, Andrew C.G., Christoph C. Lees, Arvind Kumar, Hannah H. Missfelder-Lobos, and Edile M. Murdoch. 2007. "Palliative care for prenatally diagnosed lethal fetal abnormality." *Archives of Disease in Childhood-Fetal and Neonatal Edition* 92 (1): F56–F58.

Bretherton, Luke. 2006. *Hospitality as Holiness: Christian Witness Amid Moral Diversity.* Aldershot: Ashgate Publishing Company.

Chesterton, Gilbert Keith. 1936. *Orthodoxy: The Romance of Faith.* New York: Image Books.

Cole, Joanna C.M., Julie S. Moldenhauer, Tyra R. Jones, Elizabeth A. Shaughnessy, Haley E. Zarrin, Aimee L. Coursey, and David A. Munson. 2017. "A Proposed Model for Perinatal Palliative Care." *Journal of Obstetric, Gynecologic & Neonatal Nursing* 46 (6): 904–11.

Conway, Trudy D. 2009. "From Tolerance to Hospitality: Problematic Limits of a Negative Virtue." *Philosophy in the Contemporary World* 16 (1): 1–13.

Côté-Arsenault, Denise and Erin Denny-Koelsch. 2011. " 'My Baby is a Person': Parents' Experiences with Life-Threatening Fetal Diagnosis." *Journal of Palliative Medicine* 14 (12): 1302–8.

English, Nancy K. and Karen L. Hessler. 2013. "Prenatal Birth Planning for Families of the Imperiled Newborn." *Journal of Obstetric, Gynecologic, & Neonatal Nursing* 42 (3): 390–9.

Farlow, Barbara. 2009. "Misgivings." *The Hastings Center Report* 39 (5): 19–21.

Farlow, Barbara. 2011. "Choosing the Road Less Traveled." *Current Problems in Pediatric and Adolescent Health Care* 41 (4): 115–16.

Farrelly, Ellyn, Mildred K. Cho, Lori Erby, Debra Roter, Anabel Stenzel, and Kelly Ormond. 2012. "Genetic Counseling for Prenatal Testing: Where is the Discussion about Disability?" *Journal of Genetic Counseling* 21 (6): 814–24.

Guon, Jennifer, Benjamin S. Wilfond, Barbara Farlow, Tracy Brazg, and Annie Janvier. 2014. "Our Children are not a Diagnosis: The Experience of Parents Who Continue Their Pregnancy After a Prenatal Diagnosis of trisomy 13 or 18." *American Journal of Medical Genetics Part A* 164 (2): 308–18.

Haslanger, Sally. 2012. *Resisting Reality: Social Construction and Social Critique*. Oxford: Oxford University Press.

Hassed, Susan J., Connie H. Miller, Sandra K. Pope, Pamela Murphy, J. Gerald Quirk, Jr., and Christopher Cunniff. 1993. "Perinatal Lethal Conditions: The Effect of Diagnosis on Decision Making." *Obstetrics & Gynecology* 82 (1): 37–42.

Heuser, Cara C., Alexandra G. Eller, and Janice L. Byrne. 2012. "Survey of physicians' approach to severe fetal anomalies." *Journal of Medical Ethics* 38 (7): 391–5.

Hobbs, T.R. 2001. "Hospitality in the First Testament and the 'Teleological Fallacy.' " *Journal for the Study of the Old Testament* 26 (1): 3–30.

Janvier, Annie, Barbara Farlow, and Benjamin S. Wilfond. 2012. "The Experience of Families with Children with Trisomy 13 an 18 in Social Networks." *Pediatrics* 130 (2): 293–8.

Lakovschek, Ioana Claudia, Berthold Streubel, and Barbara Ulm. 2011. "Natural Outcome of Trisomy 13, Trisomy 18, and Triploidy after Prenatal Diagnosis." *American Journal of Medical Genetics Part A* 155 (11): 2626–33.

Lathrop, Anthony and Leona VandeVusse. 2011. "Affirming Motherhood: Validation and Invalidation in Women's Perinatal Hospice Narratives." *Birth* 38 (3): 256–65.

Leuthner, Steven and Emilie Lamberg Jones. 2007. "Fetal Concerns Program: A Model for Perinatal Palliative Care." *MCN: The American Journal of Maternal/Child Nursing* 32 (5): 272–8.

MacIntyre, Alasdair C. 1999a. *Dependent Rational Animals: Why Human Beings Need the Virtues*. Chicago, IL: Open Court.

MacIntyre, Alasdair C. 1999b. "Social Structures and Their Threats to Moral Agency." *Philosophy* 74 (3): 311–29.

Marc-Aurele, Krishelle L., Andrew D. Hull, Marilyn C. Jones, and Dolores H. Pretorius. 2017. "A Fetal Diagnostic Center's Referral Rate for Perinatal Palliative Care." *Annals of Palliative Medicine* 7 (2): 177–85.

Miller, Christian. 2013. *Moral Character: An Empirical Theory*. Oxford: Oxford University Press.

Miller, Christian. 2014. *Character and Moral Psychology*. Oxford: Oxford University Press.

Miller, Christian. 2017. *The Character Gap: How Good Are We?* Oxford: Oxford University Press.

Newman, Elizabeth. 2007. *Untamed Hospitality: Welcoming God and Other Strangers*. Grand Rapids, MI: Brazos Press.

Oden, Amy G. 2001. *And You Welcomed Me: A Sourcebook on Hospitality in Early Christianity*. Nashville: Abingdon Press.

Peroos, Sherina, Elizabeth Forsythe, Jennifer Harriet Pugh, Peter Arthur-Farraj, and Deborah Hodes. 2012. "Longevity and Patau Syndrome: What Determines Survival?" *BMJ Case Reports*. bcr0620114381.

Pohl, Christine. 1999. *Making Room: Recovering Hospitality as a Christian Tradition*. Grand Rapids, MI: Wm. B. Eerdmans Publishing Co.

Porpora, Douglas V. 1989. "Four Concepts of Social Structure." *Journal for the Theory of Social Behavior* 19 (2): 195–211.

Rasmussen, Sonja A., Lee-Yang C. Wong, Quanhe Yang, Kristin M. May, and J.M. Friedman. 2003. "Population-based Analyses of Mortality in Trisomy 13 and Trisomy 18." *Pediatrics* 111 (4): 777–84.

Redlinger-Grosse, Krista, Barbara A. Bernhardt, Kate Berg, Maximilian Muenke, and Barbara B. Biesecker. 2002. "The Decision to Continue: The Experiences and Needs of Parents who Receive a Prenatal Diagnosis of Holoprosencephaly." *American Journal of Medical Genetics* 112 (4): 369–78.

Reist, Melinda Tankard. 2006. *Defiant Birth: Women Who Resist Medical Eugenics*. North Melbourne, VIC: Spinifex Press.

Reynolds, Thomas. 2008. *Vulnerable Communion: A Theology of Disability and Hospitality*. Grand Rapids, MI: Brazos Press.

Sandelowski, Margarete and Julie Barroso. 2005. "The Travesty of Choosing after Positive Prenatal Diagnosis." *Journal of Obstetric, Gynecologic, & Neonatal Nursing* 34 (3): 307–18.

Sandelowski, Margarete and Linda Corson Jones. 1996. " 'Healing fictions': Stories of Choosing in the Aftermath of the Detection of Fetal Anomalies." *Social Science & Medicine* 42 (3): 353–61.

Schechtman, Kenneth B., Diana L. Gray, Jack D. Baty, and Steven M. Rothman. 2002. "Decision-Making for Termination of Pregnancies with Fetal Anomalies: Analysis of 53,000 Pregnancies." *Obstetrics & Gynecology* 99 (2): 216–22.

Smith, Christian. 2010. *What is a Person? Rethinking Humanity, Social Life, and the Moral Good from the Person Up*. Chicago, IL: University of Chicago Press.

Telfer, Elizabeth. 1995. "The Philosophy of Hospitableness." *Philosophical Papers* 24 (3): 183–96.

Thiele, Pauline. 2010. "He was My Son, Not a Dying Baby." *Journal of Medical Ethics* 36 (11): 646–7.

Thiele, Pauline. 2011. "Going Against the Grain: Liam's Story." *Journal of Paediatrics and Child Health* 47 (9): 656–8.

Timpe, Kevin and Aaron D. Cobb. 2017. "Disability and the Theodicy of Defeat." *Journal of Analytic Theology* 5 (1): 100–20.

Walker, L.V., V.J. Miller, and V.K. Dalton. 2008. "The Health-care Experiences of Families Given the Prenatal Diagnosis of Trisomy 18." *Journal of Perinatology* 28 (1): 12–19.

Wilkinson, D.J.C., L. Crespigny, C. Lees, J. Savulescu, P. Thiele, T. Tran, and A. Watkins. 2014. "Perinatal Management of Trisomy 18: A Survey of Obstetricians in Australia, New Zealand and the UK." *Prenatal Diagnosis* 34 (1): 42–9.

Wilkinson, D.J.C., P. Thiele, A. Watkins, and L. Crespigny. 2012. "Fatally Flawed? A Review and Ethical Analysis of Lethal Congenital Malformations." *BJOG: An International Journal of Obstetrics & Gynaecology* 119 (11): 1302–8.

Wilkinson, Dominic, Lachlan de Crespigny, and Vicki Xafis. 2014. "Ethical Language and Decision-Making for Prenatally Diagnosed Lethal Malformations." *Seminars in Fetal and Neonatal Medicine* 19 (5): 306–11.

Wilkinson, Dominic. 2012. "Fatal Fetal Paternalism." *Journal of Medical Ethics* 38 (7): 396–7.

Williams, Sarah C. 2018. *Perfectly Human: Nine Months with Cerian.* Walde, NY: Plough Publishing House.

Wool, Charlotte. 2011. "Systematic Review of the Literature: Parental Outcomes after Diagnosis of Fetal Anomaly." *Advances in Neonatal Care* 11 (3): 182–92.

Wrobleski, Jessica. 2012. *The Limits of Hospitality.* Collegeville, MN: Liturgical Press.

Yoon, John D., Kenneth A. Rasinski, and Farr A. Curlin. 2010. "Moral Controversy, Directive Counsel, and the Doctor's Role: Findings from a National Survey of Obstetrician-gynecologists." *Academic Medicine: Journal of the Association of American Medical Colleges* 85 (9): 1475–81.

4 Futility and the Virtue of Hope

I. Introduction

The antenatal diagnosis of a significantly life-limiting condition instantly defeats a family's hope for a healthy child. Common scripts concerning the futility of interventions, the lethal nature of the child's condition, or the extraordinary suffering the child will likely endure may communicate a message that the choice to continue an affected pregnancy is pointless—a decision rooted in a false or misplaced hope. Lathrop and VandeVusse's (2011) study of mothers who chose to continue an affected pregnancy provides clear examples of these kinds of negative encounters. One physician told a mother that "there was no reality-based reason for her to continue the pregnancy, [expressing] his belief that she only continued the pregnancy because she irrationally thought the baby would somehow survive" (260). Another physician prescribed "a medication contraindicated in pregnancy, explaining that it did not matter because the baby was going to die anyway" (260). But there are a range of hopes that families can pursue even when hopes for a cure or extended life are no longer realizable. Families can reframe their goals, seeking "to retrieve what they can of their original hope" (Cobb 2016a, 35).

Consider a particularly vivid case.[1] At approximately twenty weeks gestation, the Farlow family learned that their daughter, Annie, had trisomy 13. As I noted briefly in the preceding chapter, nearly all of the medical literature offers a negative portrait of the lives of children diagnosed with trisomy 13. Chervenak and McCullough (2012) claim that a child diagnosed *in utero* with trisomy 13 should be considered "a dying patient" (398). The lives of children born alive are generally marked by a range of profound physical needs, cognitive impairments, and developmental delays. Given these realities, healthcare providers are inclined to recommend against active interventions of any kind including fetal monitoring, elective cesarean section to ensure live birth, or neonatal resuscitation. As Janvier and Watkins (2013) note, both the American Academy of Pediatrics and the American Heart Association recommend against neonatal resuscitation for children born with trisomy 13. Pyle et al. (2018) observe that the International Liaison Committee on Resuscitation (ILCOR) treats trisomy 13 as a condition in which " 'resuscitation is not indicated' " (1136).[2] In a study of 732 maternal-fetal health specialists in the United States, Heuser, Eller, and Byrne (2012) observe that 599 physicians report that they would comply with parental requests for active interventions in these types of case, but 394 of these physicians would actively discourage these measures. Only 67 of the doctors willing to comply with these requests would be willing to encourage active interventions.[3]

This is the institutional ethos in which the Farlows received Annie's diagnosis. They declined their physician's suggestion that they terminate the pregnancy; instead, they began to develop a plan to provide for her life. In the process, they discovered a number of families whose children had defied prognostic expectations for those living with trisomy 13.[4] While acknowledging the difficulties in providing care, many of these families expressed joy and gratitude for the opportunities they had to raise their children. Janvier. Farlow, and Wilfond (2012) write,

> Although most parents described their children as having significant neurodevelopmental disabilities, almost all parents reported a positive view of family life and the quality of life of their child with T13–18. These parents overwhelmingly described surviving children as happy and stated that they were able to communicate with them to understand their needs. Parents seemed to accept their children's limitations and to celebrate their small achievements. When children died, parents viewed their short lives as being valuable.
>
> (296)

Their stories provided a portrait of the kinds of hope families of children with trisomy 13 can realize.

The likelihood of realizing these goods was remote, but the Farlows believed that there were outcomes worthy of their hope. So, they initiated a conversation with physicians at the hospital where they planned to deliver Annie, asking whether there were institutional policies or protocols that prohibited active interventions. Although they did not want to increase her suffering or make her machine-dependent, they wanted to ensure that her treatment would be grounded in an assessment of her needs at birth rather than a preemptive decision based on deficient (and perhaps subconscious) attitudes about individuals with chromosomal abnormalities.[5] The Farlows were attuned to the real but remote possibility that Annie might be strong enough to come home. Even if this hope did not obtain, parallel planning would allow the simultaneous pursuit of the hope to minimize her suffering while she lived. For their part, the physicians assured the Farlows that there were no policies prohibiting active interventions.

When Annie was born, both the family and the physicians were surprised by the outcome:

> Annie was born full term with a good weight, excellent Apgar scores, and normal muscle tone, strength, and reflexes. Unlike most infants with the condition, she could see and hear, and she did not have the common brain and heart defects. We had reason to hope.
>
> (Farlow 2009, 19)

After six weeks of care for hypoglycemia, they were able to bring her home. She lived around eighty days after birth, receiving only minimal oxygen support at home.[6]

The Farlow's story offers a glimpse of what it means to exercise well-tuned hope in conditions of anticipated loss. Expressing and maintaining these hopes, however, required a professional community of healthcare providers and an institution willing to provide for Annie's needs at birth. The Farlows were not confident they would find willing partners in this care; they worried that entrenched attitudes and inflexible institutional structures within medical institutions might undercut their ability to pursue diverse hopes. They had to prepare themselves to fight for the outcomes they longed to realize. Fortunately, the institution honored their requests, supporting the exercise of hope in circumstances that seemed hopeless.

In this chapter, I contend that perinatal hospice programs provide a hopeful ecology that can scaffold a family's ability to exercise well-tuned hope in adverse conditions. This ethos of hope can address a family's need for meaning in circumstances that tempt hopelessness or despair. The structure of this chapter is as follows. In Section II, I describe a tension in medical practice concerning the goal of managing the hopes of terminally or seriously ill patients. Inadequate attempts to address this tension can create an institutional ethos that diminishes a family's exercise of well-tuned, or virtuous, hope. In Section III, I develop an account of the virtue of hope, contrasting it with related anticipatory emotional expressions and some opposing vices. I contend that an adverse *in utero* diagnosis can threaten to undermine a family's ability to exercise hope. In this context, I profile an expression of virtuous hope I call allocentric hope—a virtuous hope one exercises on behalf of another person rooted in a concern for his wellbeing. Allocentric hope communicates a hopeful vision of the goods available and worthy of pursuit to one who is in danger of giving up hope. In Section IV, I describe how healthcare providers and institutions can establish a hopeful ecology that can subtend the well-tuned hopes of families following an adverse diagnosis. Finally, in Section V, I conclude by describing some reforms that might foster a more hopeful institutional culture for families in need.

II. Life-Limiting Conditions and the Need for Hope

There are substantive bodies of literature in philosophy, psychology, theology, and the allied health sciences focused on the experience of hope.[7] Within these distinct domains, scholars have defined hope in diverse ways. Victoria McGeer (2008) observes that

> there is no clear or agreed upon use of the concept. For instance, hope has been identified as a special kind of cognitive attitude akin to, though perhaps also partly composed of, beliefs and desires. . . . It has also been called an emotion . . . a disposition or capacity . . . a process or activity . . . or, finally, some combination of all these things.
>
> (244)

Nonetheless, there are common features within these varied accounts. Most scholars take hope to involve a caring concern for outcomes that are construed as good, possible, and beyond one's immediate capacity to secure. Furthermore, scholars across these disciplines have argued that hope is fundamental to human agency. Finally, scholars generally agree that the ability to sustain hope is an important need, especially in contexts of adversity.

Consider several representative expressions of this view. The philosopher Margaret Urban Walker argues that hope "is as basic to us as breathing, and basic in the same way: it is something we must do to live a human life" (2006, 44). For this reason, she contends that agents have a need for hope especially "where that is all there is against inertness, terror, or despair" (2006, 57). The psychologist Richard Lazarus similarly maintains that hope is "a vital psychological resource in our lives; without it, there would be little to sustain us" (1999, 654). Nursing scholars Karin Dufault and Benita Martocchio distinguish between a particular hope for some specific outcome and generalized hope, arguing that the latter

> protects against despair when a person is deprived of particular hopes, and preserves or restores the meaningfulness of life—past, present, and future—in circumstances of all kinds. It imparts an overall motivation to carry on with life's responsibilities and gives a broad perspective for life and thought that includes flexibility and openness to changing events.
>
> (1985, 380)[8]

Given hope's importance, threats to a person's ability to exercise or maintain hope when facing a grim medical prognosis is often a focal object of concern for healthcare providers. Eve Garrard and Anthony Wrigley contend that sustaining a patient's hope "is an important element in all health care" (2009, 38). As I noted earlier, however, families' experiences within medical institutions may erode conditions vital to the maintenance of hope. This is especially the case when a patient's prognosis is bleak— that is, in those times when the hope for cure, restoration of health or function, or an extended life are no longer realistic possibilities. In these contexts, physicians must wrestle with an important tension internal to their practice.[9] On the one hand, they need to ensure that patients and their families are prepared for death. Communicating honestly about the realities the patient is facing is crucial to this task. On the other hand, they should not thoroughly dismantle the patient's capacity for exercising well-tuned hope. Hope is too important to risk undercutting a person's ability to pursue meaningful outcomes in spite of the realities they are facing. Thus, physicians need to convey a sense of the kinds of hopes still available to the patient even if cures, restored function, or extended life are no longer possible.

Sociologist Anssi Peräkylä calls effective communication of this sort "hope work" (1991, 417). There are distinct types of hope work that structure encounters between caregivers and their patients. Some hope work is curative, focusing on the positive construal of the patient's progress toward health and the doctor's agency in this process. A distinct kind of hope work takes place when addressing patients who are actively dying. This hope work is palliative, focusing on the patient's comfort. Finally, there is a kind of hope work that involves dismantling curative hopes when it is medically warranted. Peräkylä notes that this is a common practice "during the career of most critically ill hospital patients. When it is done, the doctors, family members, and sometimes the patient communicate to each other that there is nothing more that can be done to prevent the patient from dying" (1991, 422).

But communicating these realities without proper appreciation for a wider range of outcomes that are available reflects a truncated vision of the kinds of goods worthy of hope. This limited vision reflects what Christy Simpson (2004) calls a "medicalized view of the future" (439)—a perspective that shrinks the imaginative capacities of both patients and healthcare providers. Too often, healthcare providers and their patients construe the goods of medical care exclusively in terms of curative goals: healing, or restoration of function, or the extension of life. When these goods are no longer realistic possibilities, there is a tendency to communicate as if there is no hope. But there are other goods beyond these curative outcomes that can focus one's hopeful pursuit. Simpson (2004) writes,

> Opening up the discussion about what realizable possibilities for patients' futures might be, broadly speaking, as well as changing how 'success' is defined in healthcare may be one way in which the opportunities for hope(s) to arise are increased.

(439)[10]

In short, there is a tension in medical practice stemming from the dangers associated with both dismantling and inspiring hope in terminally or seriously ill patients. In dismantling some hopes, one risks undermining the vital role of hope in enduring grave difficulty; in encouraging some hopes, one risks fostering habits of inattentiveness and insensitivity to reality. This tension is present in the contexts of antenatal diagnoses of significantly life-limiting conditions.[11] Imagine, for instance, a family who has received a diagnosis that their child has anencephaly, a neural tube defect that results in the absence of a major part of the brain, skull, and scalp. Children with anencephaly typically die within a few hours of birth if they are born alive. But an affected family may cling to hopes that are completely insensitive to these realities. They may hold out hope that their child could be healed of this condition, investing energy, thought, time, and resources in this pursuit. Their commitment to this hope may have significant costs—costs that go beyond the financial investment in unwarranted remedies. Families who have invested themselves in an unrealistic hope may isolate themselves from anyone in their community who expresses concern or diffidence about their hopes. Frustrated by the doctors who try to prepare them for the most likely outcome, they may remove themselves from a space of attentive medical care. Or, alternatively, they may demand procedures that cause unnecessary suffering. If the institution defers to the family and complies with these demands, clinicians may experience significant distress because of their participation in procedures they judge medically inappropriate. Being in the grip of a poorly tuned hope may leave families and caregivers emotionally unprepared for the death of the child.

Physicians are typically sensitive to the devastating effects of unwarranted or misplaced hopes. Consequently, it is not surprising that they seek to retrain a family's goals, discouraging the development of elevated hopes for children diagnosed with a significantly life-limiting condition. They are right to emphasize the seriousness of these conditions. But underscoring the stark realities the family is likely to face does not require dismantling all hope. Pediatrician Chris Feudtner writes, "we should judge ourselves as clinicians by the degree to which we can help nurture our patients' collection of diverse hopes" (2009, 2307).[12]

Recent studies provide evidence that families express a wide range of hopes following an adverse *in utero* diagnosis. Janvier, Farlow, and Barrington (2016) asked families of 216 children born with trisomy 13 and 18 to describe their hopes for their children. These families reported that they hoped (i) to meet their child alive (80%), (ii) to be together as a family (72%), (iii) to provide the child with a good life (66%), and (iv) to bring their child home (52%). They hoped that their children would be comfortable and free from pain. One mother stated,

> We wanted to give him a good life. We wanted interventions like with any baby but if she was in pain or needed a respirator for a long

time, my husband and I would make a decision on what to do, give
her a chance, but not at the price of pain.

(281)

All of these outcomes are legitimate goods worthy of hope; they are
hopes physicians can encourage even when a child's prognosis is grim.
Scaffolding well-tuned hope in contexts of significant difficulty is a kind
of "hope work" that helps families to face the reality of impending loss
while fostering a vision for and willingness to pursue goals that are worthy of their ongoing commitment.[13] One can construe these practices as
an expression of allocentric hope offered on behalf of families in need.
They are part of an ecology of virtuous hope that can address a family's
need for meaning in the midst of disappointment.[14]

III. Hope as an Individual Virtue

As I noted earlier, the term 'hope' admits of a wide range of uses across
varied bodies of literature. I do not seek to question these uses of the term
or contest alternative analyses of hope; instead, my aim in this section is
to offer a profile of hope that can plausibly be construed as a virtue. In
this section, I sketch profiles of both the individual virtue of hope and the
virtuous expression of allocentric hope on another's behalf.

As a provisional definition, one might construe the individual virtue of
hope as a well-tuned emotion disposition rooted in a caring concern for
outcomes that are good, possible, and beyond one's immediate ability to
secure. Each of the components of this definition deserve further elabora-
tion. First, as an *emotion disposition*, hope is a settled state of character
that gives rise to the episodic expression of hopeful emotions for particular outcomes. The virtue of hope is a disposition that moves a person to
experience the emotion of hope in trait-relevant circumstances.

Second, as a *well-tuned* disposition, the characteristic patterns of
response to which the virtue of hope gives rise involve proper attunement
both toward one's agential limits and the external circumstances vital to
the realization of particular hopes.[15] Poorly tuned hopes display an insensitivity to either one or both of these factors. They may lead a person to
dwell too much (or too little) on the realization of some outcome; his
expressions and actions may betray too much (or too little) confidence
in their realization. Poorly tuned hopes may lead him to engage in flights
of fancy about what is possible. As Luc Bovens (1999) notes, hope can
be "an open invitation for wishful thinking and can interfere with [one's]
epistemic rationality" (680).

Third, as a virtue rooted in a caring concern for possible goods one
construes as *beyond one's immediate ability to secure*, hope will manifest in distinct patterns of feeling, desire, longing, motivation, thought,
and activity—construed broadly to include mental acts of imagining,

attending, concentrating, and anticipating—oriented around the realization of these outcomes. Hope tilts a person toward the goods for which he longs, anticipating and striving for their realization. There are social implications for the interior movements of virtuous hope: it mobilizes a person to entrust himself to others when these relationships are crucial to the realization of hoped-for goods.

Fourth, virtuous hope disposes a person to anticipate and strive for possible outcomes that are, in fact, *real goods*. The exercise of the virtue of hope requires more than the pursuit of outcomes one construes as good; hope is virtuous only if its objects are objectively good. But it requires more than this: given the differences in the relative weight or value of the respective goods, the virtuous expression of hope requires a proper ordering of one's hopes relative to each other. For instance, the good of sustaining a child's life through extraordinary treatments can be at odds with the good of alleviating suffering. Pursuing treatments in the hope of extending life is not virtuous merely because it aims at the good of life.

Fifth, the virtue of hope involves construing real goods that are beyond one's immediate ability to secure as *possible*. In order to grasp hope's characteristic sensitivity and attunement to real-world possibilities, it may be helpful to contrast its affective expression with the felt experience of related anticipatory emotional appraisals. Consider, for instance, the differences between a virtuous hope for an outcome p and the positive feelings of optimism or confident expectation concerning p. The person who feels optimistic or expectant about p displays a sense of security concerning the realization of p. Virtuous hope lacks this sense of assurance: the hopeful person is attuned to the fact that his hopes may be disappointed. But this sensitivity to disappointment is not identical with feelings of pessimism or fearful expectation concerning p, both of which display a sense of security about the unlikely realization of p. One may display these attitudes because one assumes defeat or because one is excessively attentive to the probability of p's defeat.[16] By contrast, the hopeful person anticipates the real possibility of realizing a desired good; he does not endorse the sense of assumed loss inherent in feelings of pessimism or fearful expectation.

This discussion illustrates an important dimension of hope's characteristic affective expression: it has a mixed valence. Virtuous hope expresses itself in an attuned construal and anticipation of the prospects for realizing an important good. This anticipation does not rise to the level of expectation because well-tuned hope involves a characteristic sensitivity to the possibility of disappointment. Virtuous hope tilts a person toward the possibility of securing an important good, but it does not move him to a position where he is overly confident concerning its realization. Attuned to the possibility of disappointment, the hopeful person's mind is alert to signs of its increased or dwindling probability. Moreover, virtuous hope disposes a person to conceiving of alternative ways through and around obstacles to its realization. Even when one relinquishes or resigns a specific hope, a well-tuned disposition for hope can enable one to forge new hopes in the midst of disappointment.

We are now in a position to distinguish between the virtue of hope and two contrasting vices: presumption and despair.[17] Presumption is a settled disposition to feel, to act, and to think that a desired outcome one construes as good is secure and cannot be disappointed.[18] The presumptuous person attends to positive signs of success, habitually failing to see or to appreciate the vulnerable position he actually inhabits. His selective attention feeds a sense of privilege—a felt entitlement to the goods he construes as already in hand. He is disposed to feelings of optimism and confident expectation concerning the outcomes he desires. There is an implied normative stance internal to his presumption: the defeat of these expectations is not merely disappointing, it robs him of something he was due.[19] Actual disappointment of this expectation is likely to induce reactions of anger, resentment, and distrust. The presumptuous person also displays significant flaws in his intellectual character. He fails to display a proper appreciation for his epistemic powers and abilities: he is overconfident, overestimates his level of knowledge and understanding, and idealizes his epistemic position. These flaws are rooted in the satisfaction he derives from the security his presumption provides; they are motivated failures rooted in an over-inflated sense that he is immune to disappointment.

The person with the virtue of hope, on the other hand, is attentive to the vulnerable position he occupies. His affective responses to this vulnerability are tethered to a proper estimation of the prospects of realizing his hopes. He feels no sense of entitlement concerning its realization. If it comes to fruition, he experiences both joy and gratitude; if circumstances prevent its realization, he experiences disappointment but does not react with anger, resentment, or distrust.

The vice most radically at odds with the virtue of hope is despair.[20] In this context, it is important to distinguish between episodic feelings of despair, which might be construed as a deep sense of sadness rooted in the sense that desired outcomes cannot be realized, and a disposition that habitually gives rise to this sense of despondency. The vice of despair is not the mere absence of episodic hope or the felt assurance of the impossibility of realizing some important good. The despairing agent does more than resign his hopes for some outcome: he is committed to the impossibility of its realization. This commitment may be the result of an unfounded certainty that all hope is lost; it may reflect a deeper evaluative commitment that hope is not worth the investment. The person with the vice of despair moves beyond resignation to the resolution that the outcomes he desires cannot be attained. He acts in accordance with this stance: the agent who has the vice of despair is resolute in his commitment to the impossibility of securing good outcomes. The implicit commitment to the impossibility of realizing a desired good makes the despairing person resistant to its possible realization. There is a kind of stubbornness or intransigence implicit in this disposition that skews the landscape of perceived possibility. His construal of what is possible reflects the narrow and fixed picture his underlying commitment affords. As a result of his constricted stance, the despairing person forfeits the ongoing pursuit of particular outcomes; he no longer seeks out or strains toward their realization. He willingly gives up his pursuit because he is committed to their inevitable defeat.[21]

The hopeful person, on the other hand, is attuned to and focused upon the real possibilities of realizing important hoped-for goods. He does not expeditiously forfeit particular hopes for desired goods. Even when conditions warrant relinquishing a particular hope, he does not lose all hope because he retains a sense that there is meaning in pursuing other aligned goods. In circumstances that appear hopeless, an exercise of virtuous hope can enable one to cling to the possibility that there may be as-yet undetected goods one can realize if one can endure.

On the view I have just sketched, one can endure in hope even if one cannot imagine possible goods worthy of one's hope. One might wonder whether this dispositional stance is an expression of well-tuned hope. It is not clear that this stance is generally reasonable; such a stance may be detrimental to one's ability to cope with the realities of adverse conditions. Entertaining the possibility of undetected but possible goods may not be appropriate if it causes one to think or to act in foolish or otherwise destructive ways. But this alone is not a sufficient reason to counsel against enduring in hope. As Margaret Urban Walker (2006) notes, "Rather than condemning hope, we might do better to encourage imagination and flexibility that would allow those who hope on meager grounds to direct their energies toward productive and pleasing, rather than painful and costly, expressions of hope" (58).[22]

At this point, I have offered a portrait of the individual virtue of hope, contrasting it with the vices of presumption and despair. In general, virtuous hope is a kind of well-tuned emotion disposition rooted in a caring concern for outcomes that are good, possible, and beyond one's immediate ability to secure. Dispositional hope of this kind can support endurance in conditions of significant adversity because it enables one to refuse the view that there are no possible goods worthy of one's hope. In conditions where no such good appears possible, the exercise of well-tuned hope enables one to remain open to as-yet undetected outcomes that are realizable. In this way, virtuous hope enables one to resist the temptations of the vice of despair. As I noted in the previous section, this is the kind of dispositional hope that is important to encourage in patients and caregivers as they face a grave diagnosis. It is not an unqualified, excessive hope in the possibility of a cure. It is a well-tuned hope that enables the person to address the realities of his experience while remaining open to the possibility of goods that remain realizable even in the absence of a cure or healing.

This may be sufficient as a general account of the virtue of hope, but the argument of this chapter requires an extended discussion of what I earlier called allocentric hope. The best way to think about this specific expression of virtuous hope is to note how hope may be expressed for distinct subjects. Egocentric hope is chiefly concerned with one's own good; allocentric hope is a hope rooted in a caring concern for the good of another. When an individual expresses allocentric hope, he hopes *on the other's behalf* for an outcome that is good *for the other*, possible, and beyond his immediate ability to secure for the other.[23] The caring concern at the heart of allocentric hope issues in patterns of feeling, desire, longing, motivation, thought, and activity oriented around realizing this outcome for the other person.

The virtuous expression of allocentric hope involves a characteristic sensitivity to the vulnerability occasioned by another's susceptibility to hopelessness or despair. Given the value of hope, caring concern for another person makes one attentive to those conditions that threaten to erode or destroy the person's ability to exercise well-tuned hope. One's care for the other moves one to scaffold the other's ability to maintain and to exercise well-tuned hope in adverse conditions. One may search actively for outcomes that are worthy of the other's ongoing hope or activate one's imagination to find pathways to the realization of recognizably realizable goods. In either case, one seeks to communicate a vision of the hopes that are available and worthy of the other's pursuit. By extending hope on another's behalf, one seeks to show that it is possible for the other to rediscover meaning and value. Allocentric hope is an expression of a commitment to the other's good; it is a way of *being for* him. One has not lost hope in the other's good even if the other can no longer see how it is possible.

The expression of allocentric hope can provide affectively charged relational scaffolding encouraging the other to endure in hope or to strive for new hopes in the midst of adversity. It can offer a supportive structure for the ability to maintain dispositional hope even in the midst of almost certain disappointment of particular outcomes. The person who is tempted by hopelessness will feel the effects of the other's refusal to abandon him to hopelessness and despair. Experiencing this care can enable him to see his circumstances from the hopeful perspective of the other. If the other sees his situation as containing meaningful possibilities or, at least, values worth pursuing, he may be able to place his trust in these hopes on his behalf. Even when he does not yet feel capable of hope, he can entrust himself to the other's hopes and, thereby, resist despair. The hopeful vision extended on his behalf may be what he needs to remain open to possible goods that he had not seen. And the relational expression of hope in these goods can provide emotional reserves he needs to maintain and exercise a well-tuned dispositional hope in spite of the harsh realities he is facing.

At this point, one might have a sense for both the basic contours of the individual virtue of hope and the virtuous expression of allocentric hope on another's behalf. Furthermore, one might see how allocentric hope fits within the cluster of virtues I map in this book. It shares with hospitality, solidarity, and compassion a concern for the good of another. But it differs from these other virtues in several ways. First, it is responsive to a distinct type of vulnerability: the need for well-tuned hope in conditions that tempt despair. Allocentric hopes offered on another's behalf communicate a hopeful vision of goods available for those who are otherwise unable to see how they can retain hope in the midst of adversity. They provide a supportive scaffolding through which an individual can come to see the goods that are available to them. The affectively charged relational support they experience in hopes offered on their behalf can enable them to endure in hope or to forge new hopes. This response addresses a distinct type of vulnerability from those of alienation, isolation, and suffering. It is a need that can be met within a hopeful ethos in which one finds others willing to hold out hope on their behalf.

Second, the needs associated with alienation, isolation, and suffering often co-occur with the vulnerabilities associated with near hopelessness. In fact, they can precipitate a loss of hope. But the person who is in danger of losing all hope may not be able to exercise well-tuned hope even if one addresses his need for belonging, accompaniment, and consolation. Allocentric hope provides a relational nexus of support that can foster a renewed ability to maintain and exercise well-tuned hope because it draws his attention and vision to possible goods he could not have imagined on his own.

Third, allocentric hope is an expression of a well-tuned emotion disposition rooted in a concern for the good of another, but its motivation is external. Allocentric hope borrows its motivational concern from one's care for the other's wellbeing. This distinguishes it from the other virtues in the allocentric cluster which are intrinsically motivational.

In spite of these differences, the needs that elicit allocentric hope, hospitality, solidarity, and compassion often co-occur. The expression of hospitality, solidarity, and compassion may create conditions in which those who are susceptible to hopelessness and despair can entrust themselves to allocentric hopes offered on their behalf.

My aim in this section has been to offer a map of a disposition recognizable as a human excellence. Given the commitments I outlined in the early chapters of this book, however, I need to point to some additional connections between the virtue of hope and human fulfillment.[24] I cannot offer a full defense in the space of this chapter, but I describe a few dimensions of virtuous hope that can ground such an account.

To begin, one ought to consider the ways in which well-tuned hope *in general* benefits its possessor. The virtue of hope is crucial to one's resilience in the face of sorrow. Given the inevitability of disappointment, this is an important trait for bearing difficulty well. As Richard Lazarus (1999) observes,

> A fundamental condition of hope is that our current life circumstance is unsatisfactory—that is, it involves deprivation or is damaging or threatening. We are concerned about what is going to happen and hope that there will be a change for the better. But because the future is uncertain, we cannot know what is going to happen with any confidence. And if what we want or need is foreclosed, hopelessness would be an alternative state of mind. Yet we need to hope, sometimes desperately, and usually manage to do so under even the bleakest of circumstances.
>
> (654)

One need not endorse Lazarus's claim that hope is always embedded within contexts of dissatisfaction or adversity to accept the general view that hope is often "a vital coping resource against despair" (1999, 656).

Furthermore, virtuous hope is crucial to human flourishing because of the role it plays in one's practical pursuits. Consider, for instance, how hope can increase the chances of realizing a particular outcome that is beyond one's immediate ability to secure. Imagine a terminally ill patient who hopes to reconcile with his child prior to his death. This kind of virtuous hope will move him to reach out to his child and to seek to make amends. These hopeful activities make reconciliation with his child more likely. Additionally, consider how the loss of a well-tuned dispositional hope can impair or damage a person's ability to act for his own good. In fact, it may induce actions that are self-defeating or involve self-harm. Or, it may lead to a kind of psychological paralysis. If the loss or destruction of hope is a significant threat to human flourishing, then the possession of the virtue of hope is vital to human wellbeing.

Another reason hope is fundamental to human fulfillment is that many of the most important hopes of our lives are those that factor in our relationships. These hopes often take relational goods as their focal concern. We hope for the cultivation of good friendships and romantic relationships; we hope to deepen in our commitments to and with others. Many of these central hopes concern those we love the most. We hope for the wellbeing of our families and friends; we hope for particular goods on their behalf.[25] And there are important byproducts of hope that are worth considering in this context. Consider the ways hope can create or sustain trusting relationships between and among persons.[26] McGeer (2008) notes that often we extend trust to people in the hope that they will fulfill this trust; at times, this hopeful trust is enough to move the person to act in accordance with the initial trust. This trust is an effective ground for relationships that are vital to human flourishing.

There are important connections between these relational dimensions of virtuous hope and the erosion of a well-tuned disposition for hope. Often there are common hopes that bind individuals together. These hopes are rooted in the cares that are most salient to these individuals. Consider, for instance, parents' hopes for a child who is experiencing significant suffering because of a terminal illness. If one of the parents loses the ability to exercise a well-tuned hope for their son, this loss may fracture the parental relationship—a bond central to their life and identity. The fragmentation within these social bonds can impair one's prospects for fulfillment within their family.

In short, the possession of a well-tuned disposition for hope is crucial to an individual's ability to flourish. For this reason, the loss or degradation of dispositional hope is a cause for significant concern. Individuals who care for the good of others will be sensitive to and vigilantly concerned with the temptations to hopelessness others experience in the midst of difficult or traumatic experiences. The expression of allocentric hope can benefit those who are tempted by hopelessness and despair. It can help another person exercise or sustain hope in conditions of disappointment or anticipated loss. Thus, allocentric hope can be crucial to sustaining conditions essential to the flourishing of others. As a component of friendships and communities, allocentric hope provides conditions conducive to the good of the individual within the community. Thus, it is crucial to human fulfillment. Allocentric hope is also a good for those who express this virtue. Care for another's hopeful agency is a way to demonstrate concern for the good of others. To use Adams's (2006) language, it is an excellent way of *being for* others—a kind of orientation that is crucial to human fulfillment. Given these other-regarding dimensions of hope, it is clear that hope on another's behalf can be fundamental to the relationships constitutive of human flourishing.[27]

In this section, I have offered an extended profile of the virtue of hope and its allocentric expression in hopes on another's behalf. But the central aim of this chapter is to argue that perinatal hospice is a common project of care that can scaffold the fragile hopes of families who have received an adverse antenatal diagnosis. The maintenance, recovery, and exercise of a well-tuned hope in these conditions may be difficult for the family. In the next section, I extend my analysis of the virtue of hope to show how professional communities and institutions can provide the social scaffolding that enables families to exercise hope in conditions that tempt despair.[28]

IV. Hope, Common Projects, and Facilitating Structures

I contend that a professional community or institution expresses allocentric hope through its commitment to and participation in a common project of scaffolding the well-tuned hopes of families in circumstances that tempt hopelessness and despair.[29] They display care and concern for the fragile hopes of others; they perceive the vulnerability of hope as a need that ought to be addressed. They devote themselves to a project of attentiveness and vigilant concern for those conditions that impinge upon these hopes. When conditions threaten to destroy hope, the community experiences these effects and is prepared to act in ways that can sustain, reframe, or recover the person's ability to endure in hope. It acts in ways that mitigate the effects of these circumstances. If it cannot alter these conditions, it actively seeks out goods worthy of the individual's hope, presenting them to the person and ensuring him of their abiding care in the pursuit of these alternative goods. Such a community enfolds the other in an ethos of hope that can facilitate and sustain the well-tuned exercise of hope even in the midst of disappointment.

All these activities are rooted in a vision of meaningful outcomes available for the individuals whose original hopes are no longer viable. This shared outlook expressed in action and concern provides a foundation of care crucial to sustaining a well-tuned disposition to forge new hopes in the midst of disappointment. As I noted previously, allocentric hope can serve to facilitate and to encourage others in the well-tuned exercise of hope. The expression of allocentric hope for those who have lost hope acts as a sign that there are others who have not abandoned hope for the individual. The extension of allocentric hope in tangible acts of care indicates a commitment to the person whose hopes are endangered by adverse circumstances. To the extent that they can entrust themselves to a communal hope on their behalf, they may be able to rebuild or recover hopes of their own. Professional communities and institutions engage in this common project, in part, by hoping together on behalf of those in need. This extension of a common hope can provide a supportive social ethos in which individuals and whole communities can sustain or recover an ability to exercise well-tuned hope.

We might contrast this with a community or institution that fails to commit itself to the project of scaffolding the hopes of others in conditions that tempt despair. Some communities or institutions may fail to display this kind of concern because they are committed to the view that the circumstances are hopeless. Other communities simply display an entrenched form of resistance to encouraging hopes for particular outcomes they take to be suboptimal.[30] A community or institution may fail to engage in this kind of common project even if many of the members within the community or institution are individually hopeful. Strangers can experience individual hope on their behalf within a community while failing to experience this kind of social support from the community or institution as a whole.

More needs to be said about social structures and their contributions to a common project of scaffolding hope. As I have noted in previous chapters, social structures frame the experiences of individuals within communities and institutions. They define and delimit encounters between and among individuals and their communities. Some types of social structure encourage and facilitate a project of scaffolding the well-tuned hopes of others while other structures inhibit the cultivation of a hopeful ecology. We might characterize hopeful social structures as facilitating structures—that is, social structures that enable individuals, communities, and institutions to engage in the collective work of scaffolding hope in conditions that seem meaningless. A hopeless or despairing social structure, by contrast, would be one that either inhibits engagement in such a project, or facilitates commitment to a project that expresses the vice of despair.

At this point, it is important to apply this abstract theoretical framework to the concrete experience of families who have received an adverse *in utero* diagnosis. I noted earlier that families may find it difficult to maintain or recover hope following an adverse diagnosis. Given the grim prognosis, the choice to continue a pregnancy may seem pointless. Medical interventions are futile with respect to curing the child or to ensuring a long life; it is not clear that they will provide any benefit to the child or the family. Aggressive measures may produce unnecessary suffering. If these are the prevailing attitudes among healthcare providers and medical institutions, it is no wonder families find it difficult to hope. When these judgments inform protocols in counseling or become encoded in institutional policies, they can contribute to a social ethos in which hope becomes unthinkable or virtually impossible to sustain. They may undercut the motivation to develop programs specifically devoted to providing care that could help realize more limited hopes.

But these attitudes, social structures, and their resulting practices reflect a narrow view of the kinds of goods that might be achieved through medical intervention following an adverse diagnosis. Even if there is no hope for cure, there are a number of important goods that may focus the family's desires. Many of these goods are viable in spite of a grim prognosis. Healthcare providers who act to help the family honor their time with their child can energize these hopes. Even when a prognosis is bleak, planning for the child's birth and the care they can provide can enable the family to cling to alternative hopes: to meet, to hold, to love, and to care for their child. Hoping in these outcomes itself can add significant meaning to the family's experience. There is comfort in the assurance that if the child is born in distress, there is available care that can alleviate suffering or pain. Throughout the experience, the committed presence of healthcare providers and supportive centers of care sends the message that there is value in persevering in their hopes to care for the child. Allocentric hope offered on behalf of the family provides a scaffolding for the maintenance and exercise of well-tuned hope in the midst of adversity.

As a way of illustrating these points, it is helpful to consider the experience of a family who benefitted from an established program of care. Claudia and Christopher Schrock's daughter, Charity, was diagnosed *in utero* with Alobar Holoprosencephaly (HPE), a rare and severe condition in which the brain fails to divide into both right and left hemispheres.[31] Only a small percentage of unborn children diagnosed with HPE will be born alive; of those who are born alive, only a small percentage will live beyond six months. The Schrock family received this devastating diagnosis, sensitive to the harsh statistical reality of what they were facing. They understood that they "would most likely never have the opportunity to meet before [Charity's] premature end" (12). Nonetheless, they chose to carry the pregnancy to term. Their physician referred them to EDMARC Hospice for Children because of the challenges they were likely to face. The Schrocks write,

> at the time, we did not fully realize the amount of support we needed, or fully appreciate the gift we had just been given. EDMARC listened to our diagnosis and asked us how they could help. As we approached the ninth month of a pregnancy (that wasn't supposed to be), we asked for help writing a birthing plan and developing plans to enjoy what few precious moments we may be granted with our child.
>
> (Schrock and Schrock 2017, 12–13)

Writing this plan enabled them to put in writing the kinds of hopes they desired to pursue in a context they had not anticipated. They did not expect to make it to birth, but given that this outcome now seemed likely, they needed to prepare themselves for the goods they desired to secure. EDMARC provided a structured process that could support the exercise of well-tuned hope.

When Charity was born, the entire team acted in accordance with the plan they had developed: physicians and nurses provided a supportive atmosphere in which the family could be with Charity, hold her, feed her, introduce her to her siblings, and participate in religious rituals. But something interesting occurred that no one had expected: Charity did not die immediately after birth. And after two weeks in the hospital, they were able to bring her home. They had not prepared fully for what it would mean to address her ongoing needs, but EDMARC was present again, providing ongoing medical care when necessary and connecting them with a support group for families with children who had HPE. Together these groups worked to support the Schrock family in providing for Charity's needs. Although her experience at home was marked by frequent visits to the hospital, Charity lived for almost three years before her death. She was a loved member of her family, a child whose life was both meaningful and good.

The Schrock's story provides further evidence that perinatal hospice should not be construed merely as a form of comfort care. It can involve planning for comfort care, but it also involves the development of parallel plans for interventions that can benefit a child who defies the odds. Perinatal hospice teams are prepared to adjust care in response to the needs of the child. In some cases, this involves transitioning a family to home care and life beyond what the initial prognosis promised. Both of the narratives described at length in this chapter also indicate the need for physicians, institutions, and personal communities to exercise appropriate caution in their pronouncements concerning a child's prognosis. Although there is a substantive body of evidence indicating that these children will more than likely face an early and untimely death, there are times when families experience the joy of being able to care for the child beyond what was anticipated. It may be unwise for them to overinvest in this specific hope immediately following the diagnosis; there are good reasons to help them remain attuned to the limited probability of these outcomes. Nonetheless, in their engagements with the family, healthcare providers and institutions can help the family invest themselves in a range of allied hopes.

Perinatal hospice programs enable families to exercise well-tuned hope even in contexts where loss seems inevitable. But these programs of care do much more than this. Structured perinatal hospice programs act to mute or otherwise discourage individual or institutional tendencies to dismantle worthwhile hopes. They scaffold an openness to good outcomes in circumstances where the medical team may be tempted to resign all hope. These hopeful structures act as an institutional corrective to attitudes or structures that promote the unnecessary diminishment of a family's hope for a diverse set of goods. They recruit physicians into a common project of encouraging families to seek and discover hopes worthy of their commitment. They promote a hopeful ecology that safeguards the fragile hopes of families who struggle to find meaning following an adverse diagnosis.

V. Conclusion—Fostering a Hopeful Institutional Culture

Families whose children are diagnosed *in utero* with significantly life-limiting conditions instantly experience the loss of some of their most important hopes for their children. Many of these families receive a diagnosis within an institutional ethos that is unsupportive of their desires to provide beneficial care. In their attempts to manage a family's expectations, healthcare providers may erode the conditions crucial for a family to maintain the sense that there is meaning in continuing the pregnancy. In this chapter, I have argued that structured perinatal hospice programs offer a hopeful institutional ethos. Healthcare providers who engage in this common project of care partner with the family in the pursuit of outcomes worthy of their ongoing hope. They scaffold a hopeful striving for beneficial care. Families find themselves within a professional community and institution that is prepared to engage with them in drawing meaning and value from the choice to continue the pregnancy. It is a cooperative endeavor that simultaneously encourages families to anticipate the realization of important goods while preparing them for the difficulties of loss. Families receive care within a community that hopes with and on their behalf for the realization of meaningful outcomes. When one considers this institutional commitment, one can see clearly how perinatal hospice programs meet the family's need for meaning in the midst of loss.

But given the current structures, what kinds of reforms are crucial to the development of this kind of institutional culture? As I discussed in the previous chapter, the first steps to reform involve changes in the practices of delivering significantly life-limiting diagnoses. Professional communities and institutions must seek to curb those practices that imply or reinforce the view that there are no goods for which families can hope. In this context, two particular tendencies must be addressed. First, physicians must avoid using language that discounts or fails to attend to prognostic uncertainties. For instance, both trisomy 13 and HPE are likely to lead to early death. Both conditions give rise to significant limitations and difficulties in care if the child survives beyond the first days of life. These statistical realities are important; healthcare providers must inform families of these truths. They need to ensure that the family prepares for the likely loss of their child. But individual children sometimes defy these odds and professional communities need to be sensitive to these possibilities. The failure to discuss prognostic uncertainties may dismantle a family's capacity for maintaining or recovering hope in the face of loss.

Second, professional communities should exercise care in their use of the language of futility.[32] With respect to some goals, such as the goal of curing or extending a child's life indefinitely, medical interventions may be futile. But this is a very specific kind of futility. There are medical interventions that can help families to realize more limited goals; these interventions are not futile. Some forms of care can extend the life of the child so that the family can hold him, welcome him into their personal community, engage in acts of caregiving, and participate in religious rituals. Although these interventions may not prevent his untimely death or ensure that they can bring him home, they make possible the realization of important hopes. Healthcare providers can communicate that interventions will not cure the underlying condition and are not likely to prevent early death, but they can add that there are forms of care that can secure other goods and prevent needless suffering.

There is an additional reason to be cautious in the use of the language of medical futility. In some cases, physicians may employ this language to communicate that interventions cannot assure quality of life. This use of language is problematic because it can express a value-laden conception of what counts as a quality life. At the extreme, it assumes that individuals with significant life-limiting conditions cannot experience a valuable life. Perhaps more modestly, it assumes that the lives of individuals with these conditions fall below a threshold such that the meaning and value they experience is not worth the concomitant difficulty and suffering. Either way, this use of the language of futility reflects a philosophical vision of the kinds of life that have value. These judgments fail to demonstrate proper sensitivity to the testimony of families who care for children with these conditions.

Beyond addressing these hope-dismantling uses of language, professional communities and institutions can do more to encourage families to exercise hopes fitting for the realities they are facing. One simple way to achieve this aim is to engage in conversations about the hopes families maintain for their children. Chris Feudtner (2009) notes that part of his job as a clinician is to ask explicitly what families are hoping for given what they are likely to face (2307). If professional communities make space and time for these conversations, families may articulate hopes that medical institutions can secure through their care. They can discuss with families the means by which they can assist them in realizing these goods. They can develop a plan of care that incorporates these outcomes as integral parts.

This approach to delivering diagnoses may help families to maintain and to exercise hope, but there are cases where families may find it too difficult to conceive of hopes of their own. The shock of anticipated loss may hinder their ability to imagine additional hopes worthy of their pursuit. In these cases, professional communities may encourage well-tuned hope by drawing on the experiences of other families. They can offer to these families a plan of care that displays some of the hopeful possibilities that other families have found meaningful. They can point to these families and their experiences as models for how medical care can help one to discover and pursue goods that they might not have imagined. They can help affected families to connect with others who have benefitted from this care. Within these support groups, families may discover new hopes they did not realize were possible. These extended networks of support provide an ethos in which they can reframe their hopes, trusting others to help realize the goods for which they long. One of the most powerful dimensions of these conversations is that they engage physicians in the process of discerning the meaning that families draw from their choice to continue an affected pregnancy. Unlike the physicians who openly question the value of this choice or who characterize it as vain and irrational, these physicians learn from the families how to see significance in this choice. And they join with the family in supporting this meaningful pursuit.

Fostering a hopeful ecology requires reforming common practices that challenge the family's capacity to hope for meaningful outcomes. But more than this, it requires increasing awareness of and access to these forms of care. Structured perinatal hospice programs provide an ethos in which families can discover or forge hopes worth pursuing; they provide hopeful structures that can support families in realizing these alternative hopes. Given the argument of this chapter, the development of these programs is a way for communities to express allocentric hope through the extension of a hopeful ethos of care. The support for well-tuned hopes is built directly into the structure of the program—a structure that enables families to find meaning and value in tragic circumstances. Additionally, these structures scaffold the work of physicians in providing care that can realize these alternative hopes. Thus, a commitment to perinatal hospice as a common project of care is an expression of allocentric hope that can facilitate the family's exercise of well-tuned hope in the midst of adversity.

Notes

1 This case is described most fully in Farlow (2009).
2 ILCOR has removed trisomy 18 from this list given recent evidence of the effectiveness of more aggressive interventions.
3 In the same study, 23% of these physicians report that they would be nondirective in their counseling for severe, commonly lethal anomalies. For conditions that are uniformly lethal, however, there "appears to be an overwhelming consensus in the community that 'non-intervention' is an appropriate approach to these pregnancies" (Heuser, Eller, and Byrne 2012, 393). For converging results in a survey of obstetricians in Australia, New Zealand, and the United Kingdom concerning children diagnosed *in utero* with trisomy 18, see Wilkinson et al. (2014).
4 In their recent study of families of children with trisomy 13 or 18 who were in social support networks, Janvier, Farlow, and Wilfond (2012) report that nearly 29% of the ninety-four children in their study who had full trisomy 13 lived for longer than one year; eight children lived for longer than ten years (296).
5 Janvier, Farlow, and Barrington (2016) provide evidence that "the single most important factor independently related to mortality before going home or before 1 year, even when correcting for all other factors, was the presence of a prenatal diagnosis" (284). Children who were born prior to their diagnosis often received care based upon presenting factors such as respiratory needs. Prior to their diagnosis, these children were "treated 'as any other child' ('full interventions') until a median age of 6 days, when the diagnosis occurred. This may have given them a survival advantage" (284). But children who were diagnosed antenatally often received comfort care alone. In most cases, these children did not receive any interventions aiming at prolonging life.
6 The circumstances surrounding Annie's death, however, raise a number of troubling questions about the care she received at the time she was admitted to the pediatric intensive care unit. Unfortunately, I do not have the space to address these questions in this context. For further discussion, see Farlow (2009).
7 For a helpful discussion of the scholarly study of hope across these disciplines, see Eliott (2005). For representative discussions in philosophy, see Bovens (1999); Cottingham (2016); Kadlac (2015); Lear (2006); Martin

(2014); McGeer (2004, 2008); Meirav (2008, 2009); Pettit (2004); Snow (2013); and Walker (2006).

8 One feature common to distinct disciplinary expressions of the need for hope is the distinction between intentional hopes for a specific outcome and an underlying hopeful orientation or disposition. For recent philosophical reflection concerning dispositional hope, see Coulehan (2011); Garrard and Wrigley (2009); Ratcliffe (2013, 2014); and Steinbock (2007).

9 There is a substantive body of literature on hope in the context of terminal illness and palliative care. Unfortunately, I cannot address this literature fully in the space of this chapter. For some helpful discussions, see Cellarius 2008; Coulehan (2011); Eliott (2005, 2013); Eliott and Olver (2009); Feudtner (2005); Gelling (1999); Gum and Snyder (2002); Hammer, Mogensen, and Hall (2009); Hill and Feudtner (2015, 2017); Knabe (2013); Kylmä et al. (2009); Menzel (2011); Merrick (2016); Nekolaichuk and Bruera (1998); Nekolaichuk, Jevne, and Maguire (1999); Salmon et al. (2012); Schneiderman (2005); and Simpson (2004).

10 Nekolaichuk and Bruera (1998) contend that communicating a prognosis in a manner that is insensitive to a family's need for hope can cultivate "false despair" (39)—a condition that may be just as bad for the patient as "false hope." In this context, they maintain that physicians ought to help patients expand their "hope repertoire" (39).

11 For some helpful discussion, see Black (2011).

12 For further discussion of the ways healthcare providers can help to inspire well-tuned hopes, see Rosenbaum, Smith, and Zollfrank (2011).

13 For recent studies concerning the ways physicians can help to cultivate appropriate hope in their patients, see Olsman et al. (2014a); Olsman et al. (2014b); and Olsman, Willems, and Leget (2016).

14 Lalor, Begley, and Galavan (2009) interviewed forty-one women who had received adverse *in utero* diagnosis of a significantly life-limiting condition to generate evidence they could use to construct a theory of the processes by which individuals adapt to the experience this kind of traumatic event. They call their theoretical model "Recasting Hope," and it consists in four basic stages: (i) Assume Normal, (ii) Shock, (iii) Gaining Meaning, and (iv) Rebuilding. These stages are not meant to be linear and movement between and through these stages is person-relative. Prior to the diagnoses, most of these women assumed that they would have a healthy child. Receiving the diagnoses led to a stage of disbelief and shock over the shattering of their expectations concerning the pregnancy. After the diagnoses, women began to seek to regain meaning by engaging in activities that gave them a semblance of control or purpose in the midst of the felt loss of control. Rebuilding refers to the process by which these women integrated the entire experience into their life and developed new beliefs and expectations concerning life and loss.

15 This section draws on Victoria McGeer's (2004) insightful analysis of the art of good hoping.

16 I would like to thank Gregory Poore for helping me to be sensitive to this distinction.

17 It is worth noting that one can fail to hit the mark without manifesting some competing vice. There are many ways in which one may fail to express proper hope without expressing the vices of presumption or despair. So, although the failure to possess and exercise hope is a failure in virtue, it is not necessarily an expression of vice.

18 In this case, I am not concerned with the kinds of presumption displayed in cases where the evidence is such that one has no reason to be insecure about

the realization of a desired outcome. In these cases, if the outcome fails to obtain, one can acknowledge one's presumption without attributing it to a vicious failure to attend to its possible disappointment. The vice of presumption, however, displays itself in an epistemic resistance to the possibility of disappointment that keeps the presumptuous person from honestly appraising his epistemic situation. In Cobb (2019), I offer a profile of presumption as an intellectual vice rooted in a concern for self-importance one seeks to satisfy by privileging one's current epistemic position. The account of presumption I offer in this chapter builds upon this account but expands the focus beyond the profile of presumption as an intellectual vice.

19 For helpful discussion of the implied normativity associated with positive expectations, see Miceli and Castelfranchi (2010).

20 For this reason, I focus exclusively on this vice in the remainder of the chapter.

21 There are times when this kind of entrenched despair is the outcome of such significant suffering that one should not blame the despairing person. Although despair involves a kind of hardened stance against the possibility of the good, the difficulties many people endure because of horrendous evils or the daily experience of systemic injustice are such that they may bring a person to a state of total despair. These lamentable cases are noteworthy, in part, because I think they point to the need to care in such a way that affected individuals might recover an ability to doubt their own despair. Communities of virtue may be able to prevent individuals from succumbing to this kind of despair or help those who despair move away from their committed hopelessness, opening themselves to the possibility of hope. I address some of these issues in Cobb (2016b, 2017). For similar observations and their relevance for the theological virtue of hope, see Cobb and Green (2017).

22 I would like to thank Gregory Poore for helping me to see the need to address this objection.

23 There are likely some hopes that target goods that are shared by two or more individuals, but the focus of the hope I describe in the following is allocentric—it chiefly concerns the good of another.

24 Empirical literature designed to test C.R. Snyder's Hope Theory indicates important connections between high hopes and academic and athletic achievement, greater physical health and well-being, increased psychological resiliency and facility for coping with illness and pain, and a deepened capacity for healthy engagement in social relationships. See Snyder (2002) and Shorey et al. (2002) for discussion. On this view, to hope for p is to hold a complex cognitive attitude toward one's agency and one's sense that one can forge pathways to achieve one's goals. Given that my profile hope differs from this construct, I cannot employ these results directly in defense of the claim that the virtue of hope is crucial to human flourishing.

25 For a recent articulation and defense of the psychology of other-oriented or vicarious hopes, see Howell and Larsen (2015).

26 See Adam Kadlac (2015) for discussion.

27 I develop these ideas further in the next section by considering how communities can hope on behalf of families affected by adverse *in utero* diagnoses.

28 I borrow the language of scaffolding from McGeer (2004).

29 Engaging in this project well involves helping families to avoid both the vices of presumption and despair, but in what follows I focus primarily on the temptation to despair. In these cases, professional communities and medical institutions are unlikely to encourage presumption; current structures are such that they will more likely facilitate resignation or even despair.

30 Some communities and institutions may fail to engage in this kind of common project but not because of a vice of despair; as in the individual case,

failure to possess or exercise the virtue of hope is not equivalent to possessing or manifesting a vice of despair.

31 For further discussion of their story, see Schrock and Schrock (2017).

32 My discussion here is indebted to Janvier and Watkins (2013). For further discussion of the concept of medical futility, see Schneiderman, Jecker, and Jonsen (1990).

References

Adams, Robert. 2006. *A Theory of Virtue: Excellence in Being for the Good.* Oxford: Clarendon Press.

Black, Beth Perry. 2011. "Truth Telling and Severe Fetal Diagnosis: A Virtue Ethics Perspective." *The Journal of Perinatal & Neonatal Nursing* 25 (1): 13–20.

Bovens, Luc. 1999. "The Value of Hope." *Philosophy and Phenomenological Research* 59: 667–81.

Cellarius, Victor. 2008. "Considering the Ethics of Hope." *Journal of Palliative Care* 24 (2): 110–16.

Chervenak, Frank A. and Laurence B. McCullough. 2012. "Ethical Dimensions of Fetal Neurology." *Seminars in Fetal and Neonatal Medicine* 17 (5): 253–5.

Cobb, Aaron D. 2016a. "Acknowledged Dependence and the Virtues of Perinatal Hospice." *Journal of Medicine and Philosophy* 41 (1): 25–40.

Cobb, Aaron D. 2016b. "Hope and the Problem of Divine Silence." *European Journal for Philosophy of Religion* 8 (4): 157–78.

Cobb, Aaron D. 2017. "The Silence of God and the Theological Virtue of Hope." *Res Philosophica* 94 (1): 23–41.

Cobb, Aaron D. 2019. "Hope for Intellectual Humility." *Episteme* 16 (1): 56–72.

Cobb, Aaron D. and Adam Green. 2017. "The Theological Virtue of Hope as a Social Virtue." *The Journal of Analytic Theology* 5 (1): 230–50.

Cottingham, John. 2016. "Hope and the Virtues." In *Hope: Claremont Studies in the Philosophy of Religion*, edited by Ingolf U. Dalferth and Marlene A. Block, 13–32. Tübingen, Germany: Mohr Siebeck.

Coulehan, Jack. 2011. "Deep Hope: A Song Without Words." *Theoretical Medicine and Bioethics* 32 (3): 143–60.

Dufault, Karin, and Benita C. Martocchio. 1985. "Symposium on Compassionate Care and the Dying Experience. Hope: Its Spheres and Dimensions." *The Nursing Clinics of North America* 20: 379–91.

Eliott, Jaklin A. 2013. "Hope-lore and the Compassionate Clinician." *Journal of Pain and Symptom Management* 45 (3): 628–34.

Eliott, Jaklin A. and Ian N. Olver. 2009. "Hope, Life, and Death: A Qualitative Analysis of Dying Cancer Patients' Talk about Hope." *Death Studies* 33 (7): 609–38.

Eliott, Jaklin. 2005. "What Have We Done with Hope? A Brief History." In *Interdisciplinary Perspectives on Hope*, edited by J.A. Eliott, 3–45. New York: Nova Science.

Farlow, Barbara. 2009. "Misgivings." *The Hastings Center Report* 39 (5): 19–21.

Feudtner, Chris. 2005. "Hope and the Prospects of Healing at the End of Life." *Journal of Alternative & Complementary Medicine* 11 (Supplement 1): s23–s30.

Feudtner, Chris. 2009. "The Breadth of Hopes." *New England Journal of Medicine* 361 (24): 2306–7.

Garrard, Eve and Anthony Wrigley. 2009. "Hope and Terminal Illness: False Hope Versus Absolute Hope." *Clinical Ethics* 4 (1): 38–43.

Gelling, Leslie. 1999. "The Role of Hope for Relatives of Critically Ill Patients: A Review of the Literature." *Nursing Standard* 14 (1): 33–8.

Gum, Amber and C.R. Snyder. 2002. "Coping with Terminal Illness: The Role of Hopeful Thinking." *Journal of Palliative Medicine* 5 (6): 883–94.

Hammer, Kristianna, Ole Mogensen, and Elisabeth O.C. Hall. 2009. "The Meaning of Hope in Nursing Research: A Meta-Synthesis." *Scandinavian Journal of Caring Studies* 23 (3): 549–57.

Heuser, Cara C., Alexandra G. Eller, and Janice L. Byrne. 2012. "Survey of Physicians' Approach to Severe Fetal Anomalies." *Journal of Medical Ethics* 38 (7): 391–5.

Hill, Douglas L. and Chris Feudtner. 2015. "Hope, Hopefulness, and Pediatric Palliative Care." In *Perinatal and Pediatric Bereavement in Nursing and Other Health Professions*, edited by Beth P. Black, Patricia M. Wright, and Rana Limbo, 223–47. New York: Springer Publishing Company.

Hill, Douglas L. and Chris Feudtner. 2017. "Hope in the Midst of Terminal Illness." In *The Oxford Handbook of Hope*, edited by Matthew W. Gallagher and Shane J. Lopez, 191–208. Oxford: Oxford University Press.

Howell, Andrew J. and Denise J. Larsen. 2015. *Understanding Other-Oriented Hope: An Integral Concept within Hope Studies*. Cham and Heidelberg: Springer.

Janvier, Annie and Andrew Watkins. 2013. "Medical Interventions for Children with Trisomy 13 and Trisomy 18: What is the Value of a Short Disabled Life?" *Acta Paediatrica* 102 (12): 1112–17.

Janvier, Annie, Barbara Farlow, and Benjamin S. Wilfond. 2012. "The Experience of Families with Children with Trisomy 13 an 18 in Social Networks." *Pediatrics* 130 (2): 293–8.

Janvier, Annie, Barbara Farlow, and Keith J. Barrington. 2016. "Parental Hopes, Interventions, and Survival of Neonates with Trisomy 13 and Trisomy 18." *American Journal of Medical Genetics Part C: Seminars in Medical Genetics* 172 (3): 279–87.

Kadlac, Adam. 2015. "The Virtue of Hope." *Ethical Theory and Moral Practice* 18 (2): 337–54.

Knabe, Hannah E. 2013. "The Meaning of Hope for Patients Coping with a Terminal Illness: A Review of Literature." *Journal of Palliative Care & Medicine* S2: S2–004.

Kylmä, Jari, Wendy Duggleby, Dan Cooper, and Gustaf Molander. 2009. "Hope in Palliative Care: An Integrative Review." *Palliatie & Supportive Care* 7 (3): 365–77.

Lalor, Joan, Cecily M. Begley, and Eoin Galavan. 2009. "Recasting Hope: A Process of Adaptation Following Fetal Anomaly Diagnosis." *Social Science & Medicine* 68 (3): 462–72.

Lathrop, Anthony and Leona VandeVusse. 2011. "Affirming Motherhood: Validation and Invalidation in Women's Perinatal Hospice Narratives." *Birth* 38 (3): 256–65.

Lazarus, Richard. 1999. "Hope: An Emotion and Vital Coping Resource Against Despair." *Social Research* 66 (2): 653–78.

Lear, Jonathan. 2006. *Radical Hope: Ethics in the Face of Cultural Devastation*. Cambridge, MA: Harvard University Press.

Martin, Adrienne. 2014. *How We Hope: A Moral Psychology.* Princeton, NJ: Princeton University Press.

McGeer, Victoria. 2004. "The Art of Good Hope." *The Annals of the American Academy of Political and Social Science* 592 (1): 100–27.

McGeer, Victoria. 2008. "Trust, Hope, and Empowerment." *Australasian Journal of Philosophy* 86 (2): 237–54.

Meirav, Ariel. 2008. "The Challenge of Distinguishing Between Hope and Despair: Some Puzzling Aspects of Hope." In *Hope: Global Interdisciplinary Perspectives*, edited by Whitney Bauwman, 11–16. Oxford: Interdisciplinary Press.

Meirav, Ariel. 2009. "The Nature of Hope." *Ratio* 22 (2): 216–33.

Menzel, Paul T. 2011. "The Value of Life at the End of Life: A Critical Assessment of Hope and Other Factors." *The Journal of Law, Medicine & Ethics* 39 (2): 215–33.

Merrick, Allison. 2016. "A Paradox of Hope? Toward a Feminist Approach to Palliation." *IJFAB: International Journal of Feminist Approaches to Bioethics* 9 (1): 104–20.

Miceli, Maria and Cristiano Castelfranchi. 2010. "Hope: The Power of Wish and Possibility." *Theory & Psychology* 20 (2): 251–76.

Nekolaichuk, Cheryl L. and Eduardo Bruera. 1998. "On the Nature of Hope in Palliative Care." *Journal of Palliative Care* 14 (1): 36–43.

Nekolaichuk, Cheryl L., Ronna F. Jevne, and Thomas O. Maguire. 1999. "Structuring the Meaning of Hope in Health and Illness." *Social Science & Medicine* 48 (5): 591–605.

Olsman, Erik, Carlo Leget, Bregje Onwuteaka-Philipsen, and Dick Willems. 2014a. "Should Palliative Care Patients' Hope be Truthful, Helpful or Valuable? An Interpretive Synthesis of Literature Describing Healthcare Professionals' Perspectives on Hope of Palliative Care Patients." *Palliative Medicine* 28 (1): 59–70.

Olsman, Erik, Dick Willems, and Carlo Leget. 2016. "Solicitude: Balancing Compassion and Empowerment in a Relational Ethics of Hope—An Empirical-ethical Study in Palliative Care." *Medicine, Health Care and Philosophy* 19 (1): 11–20.

Olsman, Erik, Wendy Duggleby, Cheryl Nekolaichuck, Dick Willems, Judith Gagnon, Renske Kruiszinga, and Carlo Leget. 2014b. "Improving Communication on Hope in Palliative Care. A Qualitative Study of Palliative Care Professionals' Metaphors of Hope: Grip, Source, Tune, and Vision." *Journal of Pain and Symptom Management* 48 (5): 831–8.

Peräkylä, Anssi. 1991. "Hope Work in the Care of Seriously Ill Patients." *Qualitative Health Research* 1 (4): 407–33.

Pettit, Philip. 2004. "Hope and Its Place in Mind." *The Annals of the American Academy of Political and Social Science* 592 (1): 152–65.

Pyle, Alaina K., Alan R. Fleischman, George Hardart, and Mark R. Mercurio. 2018. "Management Options and Parental Voice in the Treatment of Trisomy 13 and 18." *Journal of Perinatology* 38 (9): 1135–43.

Ratcliffe, Matthew. 2013. "What is it to Lose Hope?" *Phenomenology and the Cognitive Sciences* 12 (4): 597–614.

Ratcliffe, Matthew. 2014. *Experiences of Depression: A Study in Phenomenology.* Oxford: Oxford University Press.

Rosenbaum, Joan L., Joan Renaud Smith, and Reverend Zollfrank. 2011. "Neonatal End-of-Life Spiritual Support Care." *The Journal of Perinatal & Neonatal Nursing* 25 (1): 61–9.

Salmon, Peter, Jonathan Hill, Joanne Ward, Katja Gravenhorst, Tim Eden, and Bridget Young. 2012. "Faith and Protection: The Construction of Hope by Parents of Children with Leukemia and Their Oncologists." *The Oncologist* 17 (3): 398–404.

Schneiderman, Lawrence J. 2005. "The Perils of Hope." *Cambridge Quarterly of Healthcare Ethics* 14 (2): 235–9.

Schneiderman, Lawrence J., Nancy S. Jecker, and Albert R. Jonsen. 1990. "Medical Futility: Its Meaning and Ethical Implications." *Annals of Internal Medicine* 112 (12): 949–54.

Schrock, Claudia and Christopher Schrock. 2017. "A Story of HoPE." *ChiPPS E-Journal Perinatal and Neonatal Palliative/Hospice Care* 49: 12–14.

Shorey, Hal S., Charles R. Snyder, Kevin L. Rand, and Jill R. Hockemeyer. 2002. "Somewhere Over the Rainbow: Hope Theory Weathers Its First Decade." *Psychological Inquiry* 13 (4): 322–31.

Simpson, Christy. 2004. "When Hope Makes Us Vulnerable: A Discussion of Patient-Healthcare Provider Interactions in the Context of Hope." *Bioethics* 18 (5): 428–47.

Snow, Nancy E. 2013. "Hope as an Intellectual Virtue." In *Virtues in Action: New Essays in Applied Virtue Ethics*, edited by Mike Austin, 153–70. New York: Palgrave Macmillan.

Snyder, C. Richard. 2002. "Hope Theory: Rainbows in the Mind." *Psychological Inquiry* 13 (4): 249–75.

Steinbock, Anthony. 2007. "The Phenomenology of Despair." *International Journal of Philosophical Studies* 15 (3): 435–51.

Walker, Margaret Urban. 2006. *Moral Repair*. Cambridge: Cambridge University Press.

Wilkinson, D.J.C, L. Crespigny, C. Lees, J. Savulescu, P. Thiele, T. Tran, and A. Watkins. 2014. "Perinatal Management of Trisomy 18: A Survey of Obstetricians in Australia, New Zealand and the UK." *Prenatal Diagnosis* 34 (1): 42–9.

5　Isolation and the Virtue
of Solidarity

I. Introduction

The wait between an adverse diagnosis and the eventual death of the child is a time of sustained need. Families need communities who are attentive and willing to endure with them as they wait. They need healthcare providers who are available and present as they pursue desired care. They need structures within medical institutions that encourage physicians, nurses, social workers, counselors, and chaplains to accompany them as they navigate spaces of care. Too often, however, families find themselves isolated and alone. Healthcare providers and institutions seem to abandon them in their time of greatest need.

Consider an illustrative case.[1] Around twenty weeks into her pregnancy, Pauline Thiele learned that her son, Liam, had trisomy 18 along with a range of other limitations including cardiomegaly, pericardial effusion, spina bifida, and significant hydrocephalus. Thiele's obstetrician offered to terminate the pregnancy, stating that Liam was already dying. After declining this offer, Thiele made numerous requests for information concerning how best to prepare for her son's needs should he make it to birth. But all of her attempts were fruitless. Thiele writes, "Without any referral to genetic counselling or paediatrics my decisions were based solely on information retrieved from the internet and I was left feeling abandoned by the medical profession" (Thiele and Blair 2011, 1).

This lack of support continued throughout the pregnancy. Thiele's obstetrician disengaged from conversations about Liam's care after she declined his offer to terminate the pregnancy. There were times when the obstetrical care he offered departed from standard practice. During one consultation, he asked whether Thiele wanted to have standard tests for gestational diabetes. Confused and angered by the assumption that this pregnancy could be treated differently because of her son's conditions, she responded that she was approaching her "pregnancy no differently than [she] would if [her] baby was healthy" (Thiele 2011, 657). In addition to the obstetrician's failure to communicate information crucial to understanding Liam's various needs, he failed to communicate with the delivery site. So, Thiele took it upon herself to communicate these needs to the physicians at the hospital. She hoped that this consultation would make a difference to the care he would receive at birth. But when she returned a few weeks after the initial visit, she discovered that nothing from the initial interview had been recorded. There was no information about Liam or his needs on file at the birthing ward.

A few days later, Thiele's obstetrician informed her that the director of obstetrics would no longer permit delivery at the hospital. She learned that this decision was based on the fact that the hospital did not have the "facilities for full resuscitation of a baby with Trisomy 18" (Thiele 2010, 647). Given the lack of communication and coordination between her obstetrician and the hospital, the director had presumed that Thiele was requesting aggressive interventions at birth. After Thiele reached out to inform him that she was seeking comfort measures alone, the obstetrician reversed his decision and referred her to a pediatrician and palliative care physician for consultation. Both of these physicians promised to help her provide care fitting for Liam's needs. The pediatrician offered the following summary statement about Thiele's experience:

> Barriers that were put in the way seemed artificial and bureaucratic but may be essential in this litigious and politically correct age. In contrast, the only real power that seemed to emanate from this family was that which was raw and basic—human love. Given the contrast, as a paediatrician, I only ever had one course of action and that was, if possible, to place Liam into his mother's arms in the hospital with the best available health care.
>
> (Thiele and Blair 2011, 2)

Nearly fifteen weeks after the diagnosis, Thiele finally received the kind of professional support she desired.

But this was not the end of the story. Thiele's frustrations were renewed a few days later when the hospital's lawyer called to inform her that they would not honor the decision permitting them to give birth at the hospital. Given that the comfort care plan involved the use of morphine—a drug known to depress respiration—the lawyer indicated that the hospital was concerned about potential legal liability. Before the pediatrician and palliative care physician could advocate on Thiele's behalf, however, Liam suffered *in utero* demise. Thiele's story is a brief portrait of the difficulties a family may experience when individual healthcare providers and institutions fail to accompany them well. Isolation and felt abandonment add to the family's burden as they endure the difficulties of anticipating both birth and death.

In this chapter, I argue that the need for accompaniment is a focal concern of the virtue of solidarity. Furthermore, I contend that the presence enacted through the provision of perinatal hospice manifests this virtue. The structure of this chapter is as follows. In Section II, I summarize some of the evidence concerning the experience of isolation and felt abandonment after an adverse diagnosis. In Section III, I develop an account of the virtue of solidarity, contrasting it with several opposing vices. I maintain that solidarity manifests itself through an affectively attuned willingness to make oneself present to and with those in need. I distinguish this disposition from the cluster of other allocentric virtues I profile in this book. In Section IV, I show how professional communities and institutions can engage in a common project of care that manifests this virtue. And I discuss social structures that can facilitate or inhibit the expression of solidarity. Finally, in Section V, I describe some reforms that might foster an institutional culture of willing accompaniment for families affected by significantly life-limiting antenatal diagnoses.

II. Abandonment, Isolation, and the Need for Accompaniment

In their pioneering work on perinatal hospice, Hoeldtke and Calhoun (2001) note that "families who have received an adverse *in utero* diagnosis fear isolation and abandonment during the loss of their baby" (527). Likewise, in her systematic review of the literature on perinatal hospice, Wool (2013) notes that parents "reported a lack of understanding from family and friends and expressed feeling utterly alone and isolated" (379). The fear of being alone or abandoned in a time of need may lead families to interpret standard healthcare practices as isolating; healthcare providers may not be aware that their activities leave families feeling unsupported. The failure to grasp the unique needs of families in these contexts may contribute to an environment in which the medical community seems inaccessible, remote, or detached—an ethos characterized by an absence of personal support.

In order to appreciate this concern, it is instructive to frame a family's sense of isolation and felt abandonment in light of the threat an adverse diagnosis poses to a family's identity. Côté-Arsenault et al. (2015) argue that parents who receive an adverse diagnosis are often already engaged in "prenatal parenting"—a set of practices that involves "making emotional space for the new baby, attaching to that baby, and having an intentional focus on the parent-child relationship" (158). Diagnosis of a significantly life-limiting condition can undermine a person's sense that he can fulfill these parenting tasks. Providing for the child's needs and protecting him from harm are a crucial part of this perceived calling as a parent. A significantly life-limiting diagnosis can produce a profound sense of helplessness. Parents cannot protect a child whom they love deeply; they cannot fulfill tasks they see as central to their identity. In short, the diagnosis can give rise to what Côté-Arsenault and Denney-Koelsch (2011) describe as "arrested parenting" (1304). The helplessness in enacting their parental identity is a significant hardship.

Pursuing care within medical institutions can be construed as an alternative means through which the family seeks to express their identity. The presence of professional communities that make themselves available to the family in caregiving tasks can enable the family to confront both their apparent helplessness and their sense of being alone. Medical institutions can accompany families in the expression of this identity. But when they fail to support families in these tasks, they can leave families feeling abandoned and alone in their calling.[2]

Some practices, in particular, may promote an ethos of perceived isolation that can be construed as unconcern or detachment.[3] Consider, for instance, the failure to communicate clearly with the family about the child, the child's condition, and the possible courses of care.[4] Inadequate, insensitive, or unclear communication can contribute to the feeling that there is no one else who cares. This feeling reinforces one's sense of isolation. This is especially the case because healthcare providers are uniquely positioned to offer what Hoeldtke and Calhoun (2001) call "anticipatory guidance" (257) in preparation for birth, the dying process, and, ultimately, death and its attendant grief. Wool (2013) notes that many of the recent studies of perinatal hospice focus on communicating with the family, emphasizing the need to "convey sensitive information in an understandable, empathetic, and balanced manner" (377). Families desire information that can empower them to be a partner in decision-making concerning their child.[5]

Additionally, healthcare providers' failure to listen well and to understand what is at stake for these families can underscore the sense of isolation from or abandonment by the medical community. Addressing the family's needs requires an engagement that is both receptive and humble; physicians cannot presume to know what the family cares about without first listening to them. As Redlinger-Grosse et al. (2002) write,

> feelings of isolation and lack of support occurred when professionals, family, or friends did not understand how parents were feeling and provided support in ways that conflicted with their needs. Thus, an understanding of parents' beliefs and perspective is a first step in beginning to help parents facilitate gathering social support.
>
> (377)

The willingness to understand and appreciate the family's needs involves a well-tuned emotional engagement with their concerns.[6] Families will not experience healthcare providers as present if they are distant emotionally. An unaffected engagement with the family is likely to be interpreted as clinical detachment—a failure to be present to the family.

Attending well begins with a proper receptivity and emotional attunement with the family, but it involves more than this. It is also a refusal (i) to adhere rigidly to protocol without individualized attention to the particularities of the family's need, (ii) to remain uncommitted and neutral even after a family has made the decision to continue the pregnancy, or (iii) to "step back" from care. Consider each in turn. Cacciatore et al. (2017) observe that affected families "noticed institutions or policies that offered perceived nonchalant, rote, or mechanical care" (9). Redlinger-Grosse et al. (2002) note that parents who choose to continue an affected pregnancy need physicians to abandon a neutral stance and, instead, "respect the coping strategies they utilized during the remainder of the pregnancy, such as planning and preparations, maintaining hope, and normalization" (377).[7]

Furthermore, they need healthcare providers to remain with them, 'bearing witness' to the meaning and value of their experience. This is especially important as the child is dying. In a qualitative study of families whose children died within the first year of life, Brosig et al. (2007) found that it is important to parents for

> their child's physician to be with them throughout the process of their child's death. This included getting information from the physician about what would happen at the time of the child's death, as well as the physician being present or available when the child actually died. . . . Parents who indicated that their child's physician was not present at the time of death reported more negative experiences, especially if they had been told that the physician would be there for them.
>
> (513)

Physicians or nurses who appear to step back from families during these moments are often unaware that their movement away from the family may be construed as abandonment. Even when healthcare providers are concerned for the family, failing to be present can add to the family's sense that they are alone.

Another practice that can lead to perceived isolation involves the failure to connect the family with secondary networks of supportive care. They may fail to refer the family to supportive institutions in which they can have their medical needs and questions addressed. Or, referrals to healthcare providers may lead to discontinuities in care. If there are multiple caregivers across distinct institutional spaces, a lack of coordination may cause inadequate or fragmented care. In their study of families who had received an *in utero* diagnosis of trisomy 18, Walker, Miller, and Dalton (2008) found that

> Discontinuity of care was a common complaint. . . . Families were often referred to a larger medical center or a high-risk obstetric clinic for further care. Maintaining communication with the referring provider was important for many families. The continued involvement

of professionals and office staff with whom they had already established trust provided families with an open environment where they felt supported.

(14)

Losing contact with these healthcare providers can have adverse effects. In these cases, the experience of isolation and abandonment may not be the result of personal failures; without coordinating structures in place, families may find themselves lost or alone because of breakdowns in communication and coordination across institutions.[8]

There are attitudes and activities within a family's personal communities that can be equally isolating. Friends and family may fail to acknowledge the reality of the pregnancy or the parents' love for the child. They may engage in ways that are insensitive to the difficult prognosis. Families may feel isolated because there is a perceived social stigma associated with continuing the pregnancy.[9] Hasegawa and Fry (2017) observe that personal communities may not be able "to understand a situation that seems beyond comprehension, [and] family and friends may emotionally disconnect from the affected couple, respond insensitively, or show a lack of empathy, despite good intentions" (97). In other cases, families may find that their communities are over-bearing or intrusive.

Part of what it means for a personal community to be present to an affected family concerns the epistemic orientation the community takes toward their hardship. Elsewhere, I have argued that a good community must adopt a perspective involving two distinct dimensions. On the one hand, communities must refuse to see the child's life

> merely as a medical complication or a constellation of limitations that produce suffering. . . . The child may face impairments that significantly alter his life, but it does not follow that suffering is the only, or even the primary, characteristic of the child's life.
>
> (Cobb 2016, 34)

If professional and personal communities construe the child's life as one of mere suffering, they will fail to understand the family's own vision of the child's life as one that "summons love" (Cobb 2016, 34). If healthcare providers, family members, and friends confront the family about whether continuing the pregnancy is worth the suffering or if they openly question the family's choice to carry the child, they fail to enter into the family's experience and abide with them.

On the other hand, communities need to appreciate the difficulties that the family is facing. If communities engage in activities that ignore the real difficulties the child is likely to face, dismiss the parents' grief, or show a disregard for the family's likely future, the community fails to enact a presence that is attuned to the family's needs (Cobb 2016, 34–35). What parents need in these contexts is a community that chooses to accompany them in their experience of waiting for birth and death. The upshot of this discussion is that families affected by an adverse *in utero* diagnosis need friends, family, healthcare providers, and institutions that are willing to be present to and with them as they seek to fulfill tasks vital to their identity.[10] Individuals and groups committed to this work display an attuned accompaniment characteristic of the virtue of solidarity.[11]

III. Solidarity as an Individual Virtue

There are a number of ways scholars have employed the term 'solidarity.' It can be used in a descriptive sense to portray the types of bonds that characterize social groups. Typically, these bonds are grounded in shared values, goals, projects, or common goods. And members of groups that have solidary bonds usually are committed to each other, identify with each other, are concerned for and about each other, and seek to support each other. Their sense of belonging to the group grounds a kind of shared affect such that events that impinge upon the wellbeing of the group or members of the group are matters of import or concern to other members.[12] William Rehg (2007) underscores this use of the term 'solidarity' when he describes it as

> a quality of human association, specifically the cohesive social bond that holds a group of people together in an association they both understand themselves to be part of and value. In other words, solidarity is a mode of group cohesion based on some level of conscious or intentional commitment (or "group identification") on the part of members. Besides the value of membership itself, solidary groups are held together by the shared recognition of a common good or goods: one or more specific value, goal, or interest, such that members are willing to act on one another's behalf or on behalf of the group as a whole insofar as that good is seen to require such action. Often such action goes together with some level of mutual dependence.
>
> (8)

There is another use of the term 'solidarity' that is worth extended reflection. Some scholars employ the term 'solidarity' to describe the kinds of bonds one enacts as one engages in projects on behalf of those outside of one's community or group. In this context one group expresses solidarity for an out-group or other individuals by acting on their behalf, or by expressing concern for their needs, or by standing with them against an oppressor. Sally J. Scholz (2008) describes this kind of activity as political solidarity—that is, a solidarity expressive of a conscious commitment to join in "a shared commitment to a cause" (34). In short, there are normative uses of the term 'solidarity' that extend beyond the description of the bonds of social cohesion. When one employs the term in these extended ways, one is referring to potential moral tasks to which enacted bonds of solidarity give rise, or the responsibilities or obligations one owes to others in virtue of these bonds, or the kinds of goods these kinds of relationships serve.

As this brief survey of some recent work indicates, the term 'solidarity' has multiple overlapping meanings. My aim in this section is not to question or otherwise contest other uses of the term 'solidarity' or alternative analyses of solidarity; instead, I aim to offer a profile of solidarity that can plausibly be construed as a virtue. I contend that the individual virtue of solidarity is an excellence that manifests itself characteristically in a committed and caring accompaniment of those in need.[13] The orienting concern at the heart of the virtue of solidarity is the need for human presence, especially within conditions of significant hardship. The virtue of solidarity moves one to *be with* others in their need; it expresses itself in habits of intentional, attuned, and abiding presence.

It is typical to talk about solidarity as a way of standing up with those in need. This expression of solidarity involves joining with those who are experiencing deprivation and seeking to redress their powerlessness. Individuals, groups, and even whole communities may act in this way, but the virtue of solidarity is more than a virtue for engaging in specific activities; it requires more than standing up for others. Consider the fact that one can stand up for others without their knowledge or without seeking a real bond or unity with them. Isolated acts of this sort, however valuable, do not typically stem from or result in any deeper form of engagement with the other in his need. One can stand up for a victim of injustice, but in a way that involves no investment in his life. The virtue of solidarity is more than the activity of standing up for others in their need. As an excellence of character, solidarity is more than its behavioral expression.

In order to grasp this difference more clearly, one might consider more carefully what it means to *stand with* others. In one recent discussion of solidarity, Jennings and Dawson (2015) distinguish between (i) standing up *for*, (ii) standing up *with*, and (iii) standing up *as* the one in need. Standing up *for* involves a commitment to act as an advocate for the person in need. Standing up *with*, however, involves a presence that transforms the relationship from one of mere service or care to a kind of mutual bond. Jennings and Dawson write, "there is something in the imaginative dynamic of moving from *for* to *with* that transforms the solidarity relationship so that a (supportive) stranger-to-stranger relationship begins to develop, a stronger kind of fellowship and mutual recognition of one's self in the face of the other" (2015, 36). Standing up *as* the one in need is a kind of deep identification between the individuals such that one sees oneself and one's good as fundamentally aligned and enmeshed with the one who is suffering.[14] In my view, this kind of identification is perhaps better construed as an expression of compassion, an analysis of which I provide in the next chapter. Although I do not endorse the view that solidarity requires standing up *as* the one in need, Jennings and Dawson's account highlights an important element in my own analysis of this virtue. The virtue of solidarity is an excellence that manifests itself through an enacted interpersonal commitment to *be with* the other in need. It is a committed and affectively attuned presence with the other in the midst of difficulty.

Solidarity goes beyond standing up for the person in the need; it also goes beyond the expression of feelings of unity or identification with those who experience hardship of various kinds. Solidarity involves a proper sensitivity to and appreciation of a person's experience of hardship; it issues in attuned feelings for the individual in his need. But mere feelings of solidarity are not sufficient for the expression of virtue. Feelings of solidarity are characteristically virtuous when they are joined by a willingness to enter into the person's circumstances to *be with* him in his deprivation.[15] Part of what it means to be with the other is to be attuned to the felt experience of diminishment. It is a presence that is affectively engaged with the other. Jean Harvey (2007) describes this kind of empathic understanding or caring attentiveness to the one who is deprived as *moral solidarity*. It is a posture of affective engagement that fosters deep (and perhaps otherwise unavailable) insight into the experience of deprivation.[16]

In short, the virtue of solidarity attunes a person to the need for accompaniment in conditions of hardship. One may not be able to rectify the deprivation and powerlessness, but one can join with those affected, accompanying them and addressing their fear of being alone. Virtuous solidarity disposes a person to recognize those whose hardship creates a need for companionship. It fosters a recognition of those in need as worthy of one's caring concern. And it moves one to respond to this need by enacting a bond of committed and caring presence. This bond can answer the other's need for companionship in the struggle.

In order to deepen this profile, it is important to contrast the virtue of solidarity with a variety of ways in which individuals may fail to hit the mark in addressing the need for companionship. As I noted earlier, there are ways in which one may stand for or with others in their need that are good even if they are not expressive of the commitment to be with others in their solitude. Furthermore, there are ways in which one may miss the mark that are not expressive of vice. One may be appropriately moved by another's need and act on his behalf but do so in a way that keeps him at a distance. The person in need may see these actions and appreciate the ways in which others are standing up for him. But this would not answer the need for companionship; he may still feel isolated and alone in his need even as others work on his behalf. Or, consider how the fear of causing discomfort or undue burden can lead one to avoid expressing solidarity.[17] In this case, the desire to prevent compounding the difficulties a person is experiencing may lead one to the misguided belief that the person in need desires to be alone. So, a person may place distance between himself and the other because of the fear that his presence will be burdensome. Even if this action is rooted in a benevolent desire not to cause additional difficulties, it is often misguided. For those who experience hardship, the presence of another individual who is willing to be with him in his difficulty is often a great source of comfort.

And there are other ways in which one may fail to engage in relationships of mutual concern and presence characteristic of genuine solidarity. One can *stand with* or *sacrifice for* those who are powerless to rectify their deprivation without committing themselves to a relationship of caring attentiveness. One may form self-regarding alliances with those in need without opening oneself to genuine relationship or for completely self-interested reasons. Furthermore, one may align oneself with those in need while expressing an attitude of superiority or contempt for them; one does so with an attitude of disdain for those who are in need. Their activities may be consistent with what solidarity requires but they do not manifest solidary relations vital to its mature expression.

The failure to display or manifest the virtue of solidarity should not be conflated with the exercise or expression of vices opposed to this virtue.[18] If solidarity is a virtue that disposes a person to enact bonds of mutual presence and caring concern for those in need, then the vices opposed to this virtue will be habitual tendencies to either excessive or deficient forms of enacted relational engagement.[19] Consider, first, an excessive form of habitual over-identification with those who are experiencing hardship. In this case, a person may be moved to stand with those in need but do so out of a need to feed his own sense of importance or moral superiority. He perceives himself as the sort of person who will join in protests and stand with those in need. These expressions of excessive identification often fail to demonstrate proper sensitivity and caring understanding to those in need. Habits involving excessive identification with those affected by hardship are vicious, but in what follows I will focus most of my attention on deficient forms of interpersonal engagement with those in need.

There are a number of potential sources that could feed dispositional resistance of this sort. For some individuals, it may be a kind of hardened pride that disposes them to hyper-autonomy and excessive independence. They are not moved to enact bonds of presence and caring commitment to the other, because they are excessively self-focused. They cannot see or appreciate the value of interdependence. We might call this hardened or entrenched resistance to the bonds characteristic of solidarity *prideful resistance*. For others, it may be a kind of deeply rooted fear that disposes them to avoid the openness to union and relationship characteristic of virtuous solidarity. They refuse the vulnerability characteristic of solidarity in an effort to protect themselves from the suffering or deprivation it may require them to embrace. They have entrenched habits of securing themselves against threats to their own wellbeing. They do not open themselves to the union characteristic of solidary relationships because they are anxious about the sacrifice or suffering such interdependence might demand. We might call this habitual form of withdrawal *fearful detachment*. Others may simply be insensitive to these needs because of entrenched habits of sequestering themselves from those whose need might impinge upon their concerns.

These are just a few forms of dispositional resistance to the virtue of solidarity; there are likely other psychological tendencies and dispositions that compete with its virtuous expression. These defective habits share some common dimensions: they dispose a person to detach and disengage from the one in need; they turn one's thoughts and attention away from the person; they entrench one within a protective space where the solitude and isolation of others cannot present themselves as a task to which one ought to respond. Dispositions that manifest themselves in patterns of detachment and disengagement from those in need of an abiding and attuned presence are vices opposed to solidarity. The virtue of solidarity, however, manifests itself in (i) a caring attentiveness to the one in need, (ii) a movement toward the person to be with him, and (iii) a firm and determined commitment to remain present to him as a companion.

At this point, one may have a sense of the nature of virtuous solidarity. But it will be helpful to complete this profile by recalling how one can distinguish the exercise of solidarity from the other traits within the allocentric cluster I describe in this book. Although the members of this cluster of virtues are interconnected, they can be distinguished in several ways. First, one can draw important distinctions by attending to the varied needs that elicit their expression. Solidarity differs from hospitality in that it has a broader scope; it focuses on the need for accompaniment independent of the affected person status as a member of the community. Hospitality, on the other hand, focuses on the needs of the stranger—that is, the person whose vulnerability is rooted in his status as alienated from the community. A similar difference of scope and responsiveness to need enables one to distinguish between solidarity as a virtue that addresses a felt need for accompaniment and compassion as a virtue that addresses the need for consolation in the midst of suffering. To be vulnerable because one feels alone or isolated is not the same as being vulnerable because one is suffering. Solidarity also differs from allocentric hope in that the need that underwrites this expression of other-regarding concern is the need to encourage or sustain another's hope when the other is tempted by despair. This need is distinct from the need for an abiding and caring presence when one feels alone or abandoned. The fact that these virtues are elicited by distinct needs has implications for the kind of factors a person finds salient within specific contexts. What is salient to the person who enacts solidarity is the perception of a person who is experiencing isolation and abandonment. This is distinct from the salience of a person's status as a stranger, a person in danger of losing hope, or a sufferer.

Second, one can distinguish between these virtues by attending to their characteristic behavioral, affective, and social expressions. Solidarity moves a person outward from himself toward those in need whether they are members of one's own social group or to those in external groups. Hospitality differs in that it opens one's boundaries and invites the person into a space of belonging. Solidarity shares with compassion the movement toward an individual in need to address the person's need or to ameliorate its effects. But solidarity expresses itself primarily in an attuned commitment to be with the person in his solitude while compassion involves the additional commitment to take on the other's suffering as one's own. Finally, allocentric hope differs from these in that its characteristic movement is a kind of anticipatory leaning and pursuit of some available and relevant good on behalf of the other.

Although these virtues are distinct, they share a common other-regarding concern for a person who is vulnerable because of his need. Thus, expressions of solidarity are likely to be simultaneous expressions of these other virtues. With hospitality, solidarity shares a common concern for relational union with those who are in need. Additionally, solidarity and hospitality often move one to ignore or dissolve artificial boundaries between and among individuals. Solidarity also shares common features with the virtue of compassion. Both solidarity and compassion are elicited by hardships that others experience. Likewise, they both involve a characteristic desire to alleviate the hardship or to ameliorate its effects through a kind of attuned presence with the other. The virtue that differs most from solidarity is allocentric hope, but the effects of enacted solidarity are such that individuals in need of hope may experience the committed presence of another as a reason to endure in hope.[20]

Although this portrait may be sufficient to show that solidarity is a distinct kind of human excellence, the commitments I articulated at the outset of the work require me to address connections between solidarity and human flourishing. In order to address this question, I will begin by delineating some of the ways that recipients of virtuous solidarity benefit from experiencing the attuned presence of others who are committed to being with them in their solitude. The recipients of virtuous solidarity benefit from the affective experience of support afforded by the relational presence of those committed to their care. Psychologically, their presence may alleviate some of the emotional burdens. Affectively attuned relations of support can mitigate the experience of deprivation. One's burdens do not feel as heavy when there are others with one in the midst of difficulty.[21]

Additionally, there is a value in knowing that others are present in one's need. The experience of isolation or felt abandonment can lead one to think that they are not worthy of the caring attention and regard of others. Furthermore, it can tempt them to believe that the hardships they are experiencing are not significant. Individuals who are experiencing hardship need to understand that others value them, appreciate their distinct needs, and understand the significance of the difficulties they are experiencing. Virtuous expressions of solidarity communicate the following truths to those in need: (i) that they are valuable and worthy of caring companionship, (ii) that their needs are worthy of response, and (iii) that their experience of loss is significant.[22]

Solidarity expressed in this kind of attentive accompaniment signals clearly that others recognize the diminishing effects of their deprivation and that they will not leave them to experience this suffering alone. As Blum (2007) notes, expressions of solidarity thus "may contribute to the sense of self-worth or dignity of the targets" (55). The person who receives this gift of presence is sensitive to the fact that he is worthy of this kind of care and concern. In this self-awareness, he recognizes an important truth about the value of interdependence. There is a good in being upheld by others in one's need.

In addition to the goods for the recipient of solidarity, there are important goods for the one who expresses virtuous solidarity for others. First, there are some immediate benefits to recognizing how one's presence benefits the recipient. There is a satisfaction in knowing that one is helping an individual to understand that he is not alone. There is also a value in knowing that one's presence with the other can help him to understand both his value and the import of the hardships he is enduring. Furthermore, there is a value in understanding how one can sustain the person in his need for relational presence. Reflection on these benefits can foster a deep appreciation of the value of virtuous expressions of solidarity. One additional outcome of this reflection is the recognition that expressions of virtuous solidarity establish deep connections—supportive scaffolding for relationships between those who give and those who receive solidarity. These relational bonds can become crucial in addressing future needs when the individual's roles are reversed.

Second, the exercise of virtuous solidarity can increase one's moral concern for others by helping one to understand what they are experiencing. The kind of caring attentiveness required to enter into a person's experience, to appreciate his experience of hardship, and to be present so that he feels the other with him requires an attitude of openness and willingness to learn from the other what would address his needs. The posture required to be present with the other in an attuned way involves a humble willingness to listen and avoid simplistic expressions of what the person ought to do to fix the circumstances. These attitudes are crucial to cultivating a proper understanding of the other's experience and his needs. Fostering attitudes of this sort can help to diminish those habits or dispositions that threaten one's capacity to cultivate and mature in an abiding moral concern for others.[23]

Third, the expression of the virtue of solidarity issues in a firm commitment to seek the good of those who experience unmet needs for accompaniment. This kind of orientation or stance toward others is expressive of one's commitment to *be for* others and their good. One's commitment to being with another in his need answers a deep fear of being abandoned and alone. By one's presence, one shows the other that one cares for them and their needs. In Adams's (2006), one displays an excellence in *being for* the good of others. This allocentric stance opens one to a deep appreciation of interdependence.

Fourth, social groups in which the virtue of solidarity is widely diffused have an important effect in the lives of individuals within these groups. These groups encourage and facilitate greater attention to and perception of profound human needs within their immediate context. One can contrast this with other communities who lack this kind of virtue or those in which vices opposed to solidarity proliferate. In these communities, individuals may be capable of seeing needs, but their sensitivities to and appreciation of the needs may lack the salience they ought to have. And, in some communities, individuals may fail to see profound needs because their communities have desensitized them to the need for accompaniment. Participation within a social ethos that is characterized by the virtue of solidarity can shape one's thoughts, perceptions, and habits of attention such that one is better able to engage in this kind of proper allocentric concern. The enhanced capacity to perceive, to appreciate, and to be moved by these needs is good for the one whose capacities have been refined in these ways.

Fifth, and finally, the expression of virtuous solidarity fosters a deepened appreciation of the value of interdependence and importance of *being with* others. It is at this point that MacIntyre's (1999) discussion of the virtues of acknowledged dependence is most relevant. Given our nature as vulnerable and dependent creatures, human fulfillment can only occur within communities characterized by virtuous forms of giving and receiving. In communities where these virtues are present, the most vulnerable receive the kind of recognition, protection, and care that they need to ensure that they can live full and fulfilling human lives. And those who act in order to address these important needs discover that part of what it means to live a fulfilling human life is to enact bonds of caring attentiveness for those in need. By moving oneself into a space of presence with others, one opens oneself to important human goods that are otherwise unavailable. One may not be able to rectify the conditions of deprivation, but one can be with the other, be present to the other, be attuned to the other in his need, and willingly commit to accompany the other in her plight. All of these forms of relationship are crucial to a good human life and they are properly described as a kind of virtuous solidarity.

In this section, I have described solidarity as a virtue crucial to human flourishing. I have noted that its expression is important to the giver and the recipient. Solidarity is a virtue vital to the life of a community as it engages with those who are in a position of need.[24] Social groups that possess the virtue of solidarity recognize how social isolation and abandonment can add to the burdens of human life. Being moved by this fact, they act to align themselves with those in need. Solidary bonds are crucial to ensuring that those who are most vulnerable are not left alone and unaided. Given how a committed and caring presence can address the fears of abandonment, isolation, and deprivation, the exercise of the virtue of solidarity is vital to addressing a central human need. When individuals commit to being with and present to those in need, both those in need and those who exercise solidarity can experience human vulnerability and dependence as a source of important human goods.

As an abstract commentary on the value of solidarity, this may be sufficient. But the central aim of this chapter is to argue that perinatal hospice is a common project of care that manifests solidarity in the way it addresses the family's need for accompaniment. Therefore, I need to augment the sketch offered in this section to show how particular professional communities and their social structures can express solidarity for families who have received an adverse *in utero* diagnosis.

IV. Solidarity, Common Projects, and Facilitating Structures

Individuals are not the only ones who can exercise the virtue of solidarity. Professional communities and institutions can manifest this excellence through their commitment to a common project of accompanying those in need. A collective concern for this project indicates that the community sees the person as valuable. Together, they experience the hardship the person is experiencing as a summons to move toward him so that he is not alone. In communities that practice solidarity of this sort, those most vulnerable to the diminishing effects of isolation or abandonment receive the recognition, protection, and care that they need. Affectively attuned companionship can mitigate the experience of deprivation and powerlessness.

The shared willingness of professional communities and institutions to partner with families who have received an adverse antenatal diagnosis is a vital means of addressing their fear of isolation and abandonment. When healthcare providers and institutions commit to be present to families, their presence can be experienced as a source of important healing. Recall Thiele's experience described at the outset of this chapter. Thiele notes that her family experienced professional accompaniment only after they were referred to a pediatrician and palliative care physician nearly fifteen weeks after diagnosis. The presence of these professionals, however delayed, was crucial to Thiele's experience of healing following Liam's death. Thiele describes the pediatrician's engagement with her in these pivotal moments thus:

> our paediatrician walked in and with outstretched arms gently took my tiny son from my arms. Sitting near the bed he carefully turned Liam prone and we looked at his spina bifida and he explained that although the spina bifida could have been fixed, there was nothing that could be done for Liam's internal complications. Arising, he took Liam and wrapped him in the soft blanket that I had made. Watching this man gently pat my son's bottom as he sat on the edge of the bed my heart had swollen with love for my beautiful son and with gratitude to this paediatrician for his unqualified support. Gently the paediatrician spoke, 'If a baby can know stress in utero then surely it can know love. Liam knew that he was loved!' All the fighting, all the tears and the entire roller-coaster ride had been worth it just for my tiny son to know that he was loved.
>
> (Thiele 2011, 658)

The pediatrician's words, gentle care, and attuned presence communicated a willingness to be with and stay with the family in their most difficult moments of loss. These words meant more to Theile, in part, because this pediatrician was the first person within the professional community who was willing to be with Theile as she navigated institutional spaces that left her feeling alone, unsupported, and abandoned in her time of need.[25]

One can contrast a community's willing participation in a common project of accompaniment with those communities who fail to make themselves present to the family. Those communities who fail to care about or engage willingly and consistently in a common project of accompaniment or those who ignore or detach themselves from those who are in need fail to manifest solidarity. They fail to create spaces where those in need can find willing companions; they distance themselves from patients by refusing to make themselves accessible.

More needs to be said at this point concerning the social structures that are crucial to the manifestation of solidarity within professional communities and institutions. As in the previous chapters, I contend that virtuous social structures are those that facilitate the expression of virtue or correct for the expression of vice. So, social structures that enable and encourage both individuals and groups to accompany those who are experiencing hardships with caring attentiveness exhibit the virtue of solidarity. An institutional commitment to be present to affected families has additional value; it encourages and facilitates greater attention to and perception of needs for companionship along with other important needs. Communities with structures in place that enable members to be with those in need are communities in which the members are much more inclined to see the need for relational presence. They foster an ethos that structures perception and attention such that members begin to look for those whose seem isolated and alone. When they perceive this kind of solitude, they are disposed to go to those individuals and make themselves available. To the extent that communities and institutions are structured in ways that encourage this kind of committed presence, they manifest the virtue of solidarity.[26]

Those institutions that prevent or inhibit such interactions or the development of these types of interdependence fail to express the virtue of solidarity. To see this clearly, one can point to some of the structures mentioned earlier that may inhibit accompaniment within medical communities. Consider, for instance, how the failure to refer families to physicians prepared to offer care may cause families to feel isolated or abandoned. Or, consider how the failure to communicate with the family concerning their child may leave them feeling like no one is willing to support them in the work of parenting. Furthermore, consider how the fragmentation between institutions might leave a family feeling unaccompanied in the care they are seeking to provide for their children. Likewise, rigid adherence to protocols can communicate to families that healthcare providers are not interested in attending to their concrete needs. Those institutional structures that prevent or inhibit healthcare providers from accompanying families contribute to an ethos of clinical detachment and felt abandonment.

It may be fruitful at this point to contrast these deficient structures with those that frame interactions within an established perinatal hospice program. Studying an exemplary case points to the ways these programs can manifest solidarity. The Wotta family learned that their daughter, Liliana, had trisomy 18 shortly after their twenty-week routine ultrasound appointment. But their experience was remarkably different from the one with which I began this chapter. The Wotta family writes,

> We were so blessed to have the support and guidance of so many wonderful staff and caregivers to guide us along the way and help us think about and make those tough decisions. As we were nearing our induction date, we had all our plans in place. We discussed what interventions we did and did not want if she was born alive. We met with the home care and hospice nurses to discuss what we could and would do if she was born alive and was able to come home with us. We talked to a child life specialist to understand how best to explain the situation to our almost 2-year-old son. We made the decision on which funeral home we would work with whenever the need would arise. We discussed all the memory making we wanted to do. It felt like, for a situation with such uncertainty, we were as ready as we could be for all of it.

(Wotta 2017, 10–11).

At thirty-six weeks gestation, Liliana arrived stillborn. The family spent an entire day with her. They held her, baptized her, introduced her to family, made keepsake hand and footprint molds, and took professional photographs with her. All of these activities were possible because a team of healthcare providers worked collaboratively to develop and execute a plan of care. Laura Wotta, Liliana's mother, writes:

> Perinatal hospice allowed us to do most of our birth planning and medical decision making prior to Liliana's birth, which allowed us to spend all our time loving her and making memories when she was born, instead of making difficult decisions. We cherish every moment we got to spend with her and have so many beautiful memories with her. The pictures we have are priceless, and allow us to share her memory with all our friends and family forever.
>
> (Wotta 2017, 11)

This case offers a portrait of the ways professional communities can exhibit solidarity.[27] Perinatal hospice programs structure support for families in such a way that the physicians, nurses, social workers, counselors, chaplains, and personal communities accompany the family from the time of diagnosis to birth and beyond. The team engages in coordinated efforts to accompany the family as they express their love through tangible acts of care. The experience of accompaniment addresses the family's fears of isolation and abandonment in a time of need. The care they receive enables them to fulfill their calling to love and protect their child even as they prepare for his death.

V. Conclusion—Fostering a Culture of Institutional Solidarity

In this chapter, I maintained particular practices within medical institutions can create an ethos in which families feel isolated or abandoned by professional communities. I argued that those communities and institutions that promote and provide perinatal hospice can manifest the virtue of solidarity through a commitment to a common project of accompanying those in need. Those who exercise this virtue commit to being with and remaining with those who choose to endure the difficulties of loving a child who is likely to live a short life. Their relational presence provides an environment in which families can fulfill their identity and calling.

But what kinds of institutional structures are needed to ensure that professional communities offer this kind of supportive care? What kinds of reforms need to occur so that professional communities can participate well in the common project of accompanying families in their need? We can begin by considering those types of structures that may prohibit healthcare providers from being present to families. There are often barriers to this kind of care that come from institutional policies or protocols concerning physician and patient engagement. If these encounters are bound by restrictions on the amount of time healthcare providers can spend with patients or if the presence I have described can occur only because physicians depart from typical protocols, then it is likely that families will experience medical spaces as unsupportive. If medical training emphasizes clinical detachment as the proper way of addressing the family, then they are not likely to find physicians or other healthcare providers who are affectively attuned and committed to answering their need for accompaniment. There may be a wide range of external structures that frame these protocols and policies. When there are economic or social barriers to modifying these protocols and policies, it may be very difficult for physicians, nurses, and other medical staff to focus on the family's need for an abiding presence. So, the creation of programs may require challenging a culture that discourages participation in a project of accompanying families in need.

But even in these contexts, professional communities and institutions can do a great deal to make themselves available to families. This can begin with effective communication channels so that families can learn what they need to know in order to provide care for their children. Healthcare providers can discuss the condition, the likely outcomes, and the ways in which they can offer care and help to ameliorate suffering. They can ensure that there are ways for the family to learn more about the particularities of their child's needs. This kind of presence creates an environment where families can make informed decisions about care. It allows them to become effective partners in decision-making. Providing clear channels for communication between parents and the caregiving team is the first way of showing that they will join in the family's desire to live out their identity as a family.

It is crucial that this kind of presence involves the anticipatory professional guidance that physicians and nurses are best positioned to offer. Healthcare providers have the knowledge and the skill to help families consider a range of options for providing for the child's needs before and after birth. The provision of sample birth plans along with various contingencies they may face enables the family to think through what they desire before there is an urgent need to make a decision.[28] At times, these plans may help families to discover opportunities for caregiving they might not have realized were available. Being guided in this process also assures the family that they are not the first to face this kind of difficulty. Healthcare providers communicate to them that they are walking with them as advocates and allies in care. This frees the family to focus their energies on being fully present in the care of their child.

Additionally, medical staff are well-positioned to ease the family's worries about providing care for their fragile children at birth. Nurses can help the family to hold and to care for the child. They can allay fears about being unable to protect the child from pain or suffering. They can celebrate the opportunity the family has to be with the child and to express their love. Their professional knowledge of the dying process can help the family to learn what it will be like to be with the child as he dies. Finally, medical staff, counselors, chaplains, and social workers can help the family to frame conversations with their family and friends about the nature of this experience, their expectations, and how to be present to them. The consistent willingness to provide this kind of support from the diagnosis through death communicates a readiness to accompany the family.

Anticipatory guidance needs to be joined with structures for coordinating care across institutional spaces. Structured programs in perinatal hospice can manifest solidarity through the efforts of a designated coordinator who works with obstetricians, the hospital or birthing center, the NICU, and other support agencies to ensure the family experiences seamless and uninterrupted care. After diagnosis and the decision to continue the pregnancy, the coordinator can meet with the family, listen to their concerns, answer questions, discuss the range of options other families have pursued, and help them to consider potential forms of care they may not have considered. Even the knowledge that other families have had similar experiences and benefitted from particular forms of care can impart to the family the sense that they are not alone. It can assure them that the professional community has also been present to others in relevantly similar contexts. They can entrust themselves to those involved in their care knowing that they have walked with other families and been with them in their time of dire need.[29] Furthermore, in well-organized programs, the coordinator ensures effective communication between and among institutions so that the family does not have to worry that their needs will go unaddressed. This relieves the family of the difficult work of crafting an *ad hoc* plan in the midst of their emotional trauma. The coordinated care made possible through organized systems can help the family to trust that all of those invested in their care are working toward a common goal.

Finally, structured programs in perinatal hospice may help to address some of the limitations of a family's personal community. There are many who feel abandoned by their friends and families. Even when they are not left alone, family and friends may not be able to grasp what they are experiencing. Given these realities, it is important that affected families have access to counselors, support groups, or other forms of social support. These social support communities may offer a kind of accompaniment that parents' personal communities are unable to extend. Well-organized perinatal hospice programs can provide information to families about others who have been in relevantly similar circumstances; they can ensure that families receive information about these extended networks of social support.[30] Social structures connecting families to these groups is itself a facilitating structure that expresses virtue.

One of the central needs of families who have received an adverse diagnosis is the need to be accompanied as they seek to fulfill their calling as parents. They need personal and professional communities to be with them, to participate in the project of completing tasks vital to their identity as a family. Too often families find themselves alone, isolated, and without the supportive care of those who are attuned to their needs. Structured perinatal hospice programs offer an ethos of caring accompaniment—a system of support where families can enjoy the presence of healthcare providers who enter into their experience and walk with them. These programs of care bring families into a space where they can feel the abiding and attuned presence of others who help them to fulfill their roles as parents. A system of support that moves professional communities and institutions to be present, attuned, and committed to these families realizes an important good: it addresses the family's need for accompaniment. Thus, the promotion and provision of perinatal hospice manifests the virtue of solidarity.

Notes

1 For discussion of this case, see Thiele (2010, 2011); Thiele and Blair (2011); Thiele, Berg, and Farlow (2013).
2 In this chapter, I focus on the ways healthcare providers can support the family's efforts to honor, celebrate, and value the ongoing life of their child. Solidarity is also crucial to addressing the family's bereavement care. I address the need for consolation in grief in the next chapter. Although I focus on the virtue of compassion, it should be clear that consolation also involves the expression of solidarity with the family. For discussions of connections between virtues with an allocentric focus, see Gulliford and Roberts (2018).
3 Coulehan (2009) argues that, "[in] both theory and practice, modern medicine focuses primarily on detachment as the proper response to suffering. The terms 'clinical distance' and 'detached concern' are also used, especially the latter" (592). He contends that there are two primary reasons for this stance. First, physicians assume that this kind of detachment is crucial to avoiding burnout or fatigue. Second, they assume that "[e]motional vulnerability impairs medical performance, and strong attachment (or repulsion) greatly impairs doctoring" (593). Coulehan notes that neither of these claims enjoys broad empirical support.
4 In a recent study, Côté-Arsenault and Denney-Koelsch (2016) found that all surveyed families sought out additional information concerning their children. Although families generally desire clear and honest communication about their child's condition, they may have distinct types of information-seeking behaviors related to their diverging coping styles. Thus, healthcare providers need to demonstrate sensitivity to these distinct types of need and coping styles. For a discussion of the distinct types of information need and their connections to varied coping styles, see Lalor, Begley, and Galavan (2012).
5 See Gaucher and Payot (2016) for discussion of empowerment as one of the key desires mothers express as they prepare for neonatology consultations.
6 For further discussion of the need for empathic engagement, see Lefkowits et al. (2016) and Walker, Miller, and Dalton (2008).
7 Too often, however, families do not experience this kind of support. The professional community expresses a neutrality that can be invalidating. Some wonder whether these actions were "the result of liability concerns"

(Redlinger-Grosse 2002, 375). This concern for legal liability was explicitly mentioned in Thiele's case discussed previously.

8 For further discussion of the effects of fragmented care within institutions, see Catlin and Carter (2002); Côté-Arsenault and Denney-Koelsch (2011); and Kenner, Press, and Ryan (2015).

9 See Côté-Arsenault and Denney-Koelsch (2011) for discussions of "social stigma" in the context of adverse *in utero* diagnoses. For further discussion of isolation and abandonment within personal communities, see Hickerton et al. (2012).

10 For evidence of the value of social support for coping, see Horsch, Brooks, and Fletcher (2013). For further evidence concerning the importance of social support following perinatal loss, see Kavanaugh, Trier, and Korzec (2004).

11 Millstein (2005) develops an account of integrative care that focuses on both "being with" and "doing for" families in these contexts. For reflection on an active, attuned presence with others within the context of nursing care, see Swanson (1993).

12 For discussion of uses of the term 'solidarity' to describe the qualities of social bonds within social groups and communities, see Blum (2007); Rehg (2007); Shelby (2005, 67–72); and Scholz (2015).

13 There are some connections between my analysis and the conception of the virtue of solidarity in Roman Catholic social teaching. For further discussion, see Pope John Paul II's (1987) encyclical letter *Sollicitudo rei socialis*. Also, see Clark (2014a, 2014b) and Beyer (2014). But the Catholic view grounds solidarity in a theological framework. Given my aim of developing a virtue-based defense of perinatal hospice that is theologically neutral, my analysis of solidarity cannot rest on the same foundations. For additional works informing my following virtue-theoretic discussion, see Byerly and Byerly (2016); Harvey (2007); Thalos (2012); and Tsai (2018).

14 For further discussion, see Jennings (2015). For an application of this framework to the question of prenatal screening for Down Syndrome, see Gabriel (2017).

15 Prainsack and Buyx (2012) argue that mere feelings of solidarity, or motivations grounded in such feelings, are not sufficient for genuine solidarity. Solidarity, on their view, consists in "*shared practices reflecting a collective commitment to carry 'costs' (financial, social, emotional, or otherwise) to assist others*" (346). Thus, mere expression of feelings of solidarity are not enough; one must engage in activities ordered to shoulder the burdens of others on their behalf. For further discussions of solidarity in bioethics, see Gunson (2009).

16 Stephen Darwall's (2011) discussion of the notion of "being with" may be helpful in this context. Darwall offers an account of what it means for two (or more) individuals to relate to each other in a way that they construe themselves as being together with each other. "Being with" is a technical notion meant to involve a shared emotional, perceptual, and spiritual experience of togetherness. This isn't exclusively a function of personal relationships. Rather, it is a form of "mutual *relating*" (6). Being with another person involves a willingness to share access to oneself with the other. It involves a mutual receptivity, openness, and responsiveness to the other.

17 I am grateful to Gregory Poore for suggesting this possibility as a kind of *misguided beneficent distance*.

18 Meghan Clark (2014b) borrows an Aristotelian approach to characterizing solidarity as theological virtue. She maintains that the virtue of solidarity lies in a mean between excess and deficiency. Importantly, solidarity occupies a

place between distinct types of vice—vices that can manifest themselves in individuals, groups, or even nations. One can contrast the virtue of solidarity with excessive individualism, on the one hand, and with collectivism, on the other hand. Excessive individualism assumes "that human persons are fundamentally isolated, atomized individuals or blank slates. Under these sets of vices, human persons are individuals by nature and social or interdependent by choice" (2014b, 32). Collectivism involves a subsumption, or erasure, of the individual within a community or a collective. In this way, the good of the individual is sacrificed to the good of the whole. But Clark contends that this is inconsistent with the *telos* of solidarity. She writes, "the virtue of solidarity involves a firm and persevering determination to both individual dignity and the integrity of communities. Neither the individual nor the common good can be eliminated or sacrificed in solidarity as directed towards its proper end" (2014b, 31).

19 In discussing the virtue of hospitality, I argued that vices of excess are likely less common than vices of deficient regard for the stranger. Arguably, this is true with respect to vices that oppose solidarity. Excessive expressions of relational presence with a person experiencing hardship are likely less common that deficient expressions of relational presence. Thus, I focus primarily on vices of deficiency.

20 See Wrigley (2019) for a recent discussion of connections between hope and solidarity.

21 In her discussion of living with incurable disease and disability, S. Kay Toombs (2018) offers a sensitive account of the value of interdependence both for those who give care and for those who receive care. Unfortunately, I lack the space to address her discussion at length.

22 I address this third point more fully in Chapter 6 and its focus on compassionate responses to the family's experience of deep grief.

23 Bommarito (2016) notes that private expressions of solidarity can have similar effects, enabling us to "sharpen, sustain, strengthen, and clarify our concern for others. It may sharpen our concern by directing an abstract or general concern towards real, particular people" (453).

24 This discussion aligns well with MacIntyre's (1999) discussion of the virtues of acknowledged dependence. MacIntyre does not make specific reference to a virtue of solidarity, but it is clear that his central focus is on the forms of interdependence crucial to human fulfillment. One might argue that the type of community MacIntyre is describing is one characterized by solidarity—that is, a community in which the members make themselves present to each other in reciprocal belonging.

25 In this context, one might argue that the institutional spaces displayed inhospitality to the Theiles and the pediatrician's actions were expressive of the virtue of hospitality in welcoming them into a space of care. This illustrates the claim I have made throughout this work that one action can simultaneously manifest multiple virtues. The pediatrician expresses solidarity in his willingness to be with the family and to guide them through the final moments with the family. He did not just invite them to receive care; he made himself available to them so that they knew they were not alone.

26 Although they employ an account of solidarity distinct from my own, Prainsack and Buyx (2012) have explicitly discussed the institutionalization of solidarity. They contend that solidarity can be institutionalized through the display of "*a collective commitment to carry costs to assist others (who are all linked by means of a shared situation or cause)*" (347). A coordinated and collective commitment to shouldering the burdens of others can become

a fundamental feature of the ways in which particular institutions operate together to address needs. They write, "This approach regards solidarity primarily as something that is enacted at the interpersonal and communal level, and that—to the extent that it becomes normative—can solidify into informal as well as formal contractual and legal arrangements" (2012, 349).

27 For a similar case study accompanied by helpful supporting materials for the construction of a birth and care plan, see Roush et al. (2007).

28 For discussion of birth plans, see Catlin and Carter (2002) and English and Hessler (2013).

29 I'd like to thank Gregory Poore for helping me to see the need to highlight the effects of these practices in ensuring bonds of solidarity between professional communities and an affected family.

30 For further discussion of social support groups in these contexts, see Cope et al. (2015); Côté-Arsenault and Freije (2004); Hickerton et al. (2012); and Janvier, Farlow, and Wilfond (2012).

References

Adams, Robert. 2006. *A Theory of Virtue: Excellence in Being for the Good.* Oxford: Clarendon Press.

Beyer, Gerald J. 2014. "The Meaning of Solidarity in Catholic Social Teaching." *Political Theology* 15 (1): 7–25.

Blum, Lawrence. 2007. "Three Kinds of Race-Related Solidarity." *Journal of Social Philosophy* 38 (1): 53–72.

Bommarito, Nicolas. 2016. "Private Solidarity." *Ethical Theory and Moral Practice* 19 (2): 445–55.

Brosig, C.L., R.L. Pierucci, M.J. Kupst, and S.R. Leuthner. 2007. "Infant End-of-Life Care: The Parents' Perspective." *Journal of Perinatology* 27 (8): 510–16.

Byerly, T. Ryan and Meghan Byerly. 2016. "Collective Virtue." *The Journal of Value Inquiry* 50 (1): 33–50.

Cacciatore, Joanne, Kara Thieleman, Angela S. Lieber, Cybele Blood, and Rachel Goldman. 2017. "The Long Road to Farewell: The Needs of Families with Dying Children." *OMEGA-Journal of Death and Dying.* 0030222817697418.

Catlin, Anita and Brian Carter. 2002. "Creation of a Neonatal End-of-Life Palliative Care Protocol." *Journal of Perinatology* 22 (3): 184–95.

Clark, Meghan J. 2014a. *The Vision of Catholic Social Thought: The Virtue of Solidarity and the Praxis of Human Rights.* Minneapolis: Fortress Press.

Clark, Meghan J. 2014b. "Anatomy of a Social Virtue: Solidarity and Corresponding Vices." *Political Theology* 15 (1): 26–39.

Cobb, Aaron D. 2016. "Acknowledged Dependence and the Virtues of Perinatal Hospice." *The Journal of Medicine and Philosophy: A Forum for Bioethics and Philosophy of Medicine* 41 (1): 25–40.

Cope, Heidi, Melanie E. Garrett, Simon Gregory, and Allison Ashley-Koch. 2015. "Pregnancy Continuation and Organizational Religious Activity Following prenatal Diagnosis of a Lethal Fetal Defect are Associated with Improved Psychological Outcome." *Prenatal Diagnosis* 35 (8): 761–68.

Côté-Arsenault, Denise and Erin Denney-Koelsch. 2011. "'My Baby is a Person': Parents' Experiences with Life-Threatening Fetal Diagnosis." *Journal of Palliative Medicine* 14 (12): 1302–8.

Côté-Arsenault, Denise and Erin Denney-Koelsch. 2016. "'Have No Regrets': Parents' Experiences and Developmental Tasks in Pregnancy with a Lethal Fetal Diagnosis." *Social Science & Medicine* 154: 100–9.

Côté-Arsenault, Denise and Marsha Mason Freije. 2004. "Support Groups Helping Women Through Pregnancies After Loss." *Western Journal of Nursing Research* 26 (6): 650–70.

Côté-Arsenault, Denise, Heidi Krowchuk, Wendasha Jenkins Hall, and Erin Denney-Koelsch. 2015. "What Want What's Best for Our Baby: Prenatal Parenting of Babies with Lethal Conditions." *Journal of Prenatal & Perinatal Psychology & Health: APPPAH* 29 (3): 157–76.

Coulehan, Jack. 2009. "Compassionate Solidarity: Suffering, Poetry, and Medicine." *Perspectives in Biology and Medicine* 52 (4): 585–603.

Darwall, Stephen. 2011. "Being With." *Southern Journal of Philosophy* 49 (s1): 4–24.

English, Nancy K. and Karen L. Hessler. 2013. "Prenatal Birth Planning for Families of the Imperiled Newborn." *Journal of Obstetric, Gynecologic, & Neonatal Nursing* 42 (3): 390–9.

Gabriel, Jazmine. 2017. "Zooming Out: Solidarity in the Moral Imagination of Genetic Counseling." In *Reproductive Ethics*, edited by L. Campo-Engelstein, and P. Burcher, 7–25. New York: Springer.

Gaucher, Nathalie and Antoine Payot. 2016. "From Powerlessness to Empowerment: Mothers Expect More Information from the Prenatal Consultation for Preterm Labour." *Paediatrics & Child Health* 16 (10): 638–42.

Gulliford, Liz and Robert C. Roberts. 2018. "Exploring the 'Unity' of the Virtues: The Case of an Allocentric Quintet." *Theory & Psychology* 28 (2): 208–26.

Gunson, Darryl. 2009. "Solidarity and the Universal Declaration on Bioethics and Human Rights." *Journal of Medicine and Philosophy* 34 (3): 241–60.

Harvey, Jean. 2007. "Moral Solidarity and Empathic Understanding: The Moral Value and Scope of the Relationship." *Journal of Social Philosophy* 38 (1): 22–37.

Hasegawa, Susan L. and Jessica T. Fry. 2017. "Moving Toward a Shared Process: The Impact of Parent Experiences on Perinatal Palliative Care." *Seminars in Perinatology* 41 (2): 95–100.

Hickerton, Chriselle L., MaryAnne Aitken, Jan Hodgson, and Martin B. Delatycki. 2012. "Did You Find That Out in Time?": New Life Trajectories of Parents Who Choose to Continue a Pregnancy Where a Genetic Disorder is Diagnosed or Likely." *American Journal of Medical Genetics Part A* 158 (2): 373–83.

Hoeldtke, Nathan J. and Byron C. Calhoun. 2001. "Perinatal Hospice." *American Journal of Obstetrics and Gynecology* 185 (3): 525–9.

Horsch, Antje, Chloe Brooks, and Helen Fletcher. 2013. "Maternal Coping, Appraisals and Adjustment Following Diagnosis of Fetal Anomaly." *Prenatal Diagnosis* 33 (12): 1137–45.

Janvier, Annie, Barbara Farlow, and Benjamin S. Wilfond. 2012. "The Experience of Families with Children with Trisomy 13 an 18 in Social Networks." *Pediatrics* 130 (2): 293–8.

Jennings, Bruce and Agnus Dawson. 2015. "Solidarity in the Moral Imagination of Bioethics." *Hastings Center Report* 45 (5): 31–8.

Jennings, Bruce. 2015. "Relational Liberty Revisited: Membership Solidarity and a Public Health Ethics of Place." *Public Health Ethics* 8 (1): 7–17.

Kavanaugh, Karen, Darcie Trier, and Michelle Korzec. 2004. "Social Support Following Perinatal Loss." *Journal of Family Nursing* 10 (1): 70–92.

Kenner, C., J. Press and D. Ryan. 2015. "Recommendations for Palliative and Bereavement Care in the NICU: A Family-Centered Integrative Approach." *Journal of Perinatology* 35 (S1): S19-S23.

Lalor, Joan G., Cecily M. Begley, and Eoin Galavan. 2012. "A Grounded Theory Study of Information Preference and Coping Styles Following Antenatal Diagnosis of Foetal Abnormality." *Journal of Advanced Nursing* 64 (2): 185–94.

Lefkowits, Carolyn and Caroline Solomon. 2016. "Palliative Care in Obstetrics and Gynecology." *Obstetrics & Gynecology* 128 (6): 1403–20.

MacIntyre, Alasdair C. 1999. *Dependent Rational Animals: Why Human Beings Need the Virtues*. Chicago, IL: Open Court.

Millstein, Jay. 2005. "A Paradigm of Integrative Care: Healing with Curing Throughout Life, 'Being With' and 'Doing To'." *Journal of Perinatology* 25 (9): 563–8.

Paul II, Pope John. 1987. *Sollicitudo rei socialis*. http://w2.vatican.va/content/john-paul-ii/en/encyclicals/documents/hf_jp-ii_enc_30121987_sollicitudo-rei-socialis.html (accessed May 31, 2018).

Prainsack, Barbara and Alena Buyx. 2012. "Solidarity in Contemporary Bioethics—Towards a New Approach." *Bioethics* 26 (7): 343–50.

Redlinger-Grosse, Krista, Barbara A. Bernhardt, Kate Berg, Maximilian Muenke, and Barbara B. Biesecker. 2002. "The Decision to Continue: The Experiences and Needs of Parents Who Receive a Prenatal Diagnosis of Holoprosencephaly." *American Journal of Medical Genetics* 112 (4): 369–78.

Rehg, William. 2007. "Solidarity and the Common Good: An Analytic Framework." *Journal of Social Philosophy* 38 (1): 7–21.

Roush, Alana, Peggy Sullivan, Rhonda Cooper, and Judith W. McBride. 2007. "Perinatal Hospice." *Newborn and Infant Nursing Reviews* 7 (4): 216–21.

Scholz, Sally J. 2008. *Political Solidarity*. University Park: Penn State Press.

Scholz, Sally J. 2015. "Seeking Solidarity." *Philosophy Compass* 10 (10): 725–35.

Shelby, Tommie. 2005. *We Who Are Dark: The Philosophical Foundations of Black Solidarity*. Cambridge, MA: Harvard University Press.

Swanson, Kristen M. 1993. "Nursing as Informed Caring for the Well-Being of Others." *Journal of Nursing Scholarship* 25 (4): 352–7.

Thalos, Mariam. 2012. "Solidarity: A Motivational Conception." *Philosophical Papers* 41 (1): 57–95.

Thiele, Pauline and Simon Blair. 2011. "Destined to Die." *BMJ* 343: d3625.

Thiele, Pauline, Siri Fuglem Berg, and Barbara Farlow. 2013. "More Than a Diagnosis." *Acta Paediatrica* 102 (12): 1127–9.

Thiele, Pauline. 2010. "He Was My Son, Not a Dying Baby." *Journal of Medical Ethics* 36 (11): 646–7.

Thiele, Pauline. 2011. "Going Against the Grain: Liam's Story." *Journal of Paediatrics and Child Health* 47 (9): 656–8.

Toombs, S. Kay. 2018. *How Then Should We Die? Two Opposing Responses to the Challenges of Suffering and Death*. Elm Mott, TX: Colloquium Press.

Tsai, George. 2018. "The Virtue of Being Supportive." *Pacific Philosophical Quarterly* 99 (2): 317–42.

Walker, L.V., V.J. Miller, and V.K. Dalton. 2008. "The Health-Care Experiences of Families Given the Prenatal Diagnosis of Trisomy 18." *Journal of Perinatology* 28 (1): 12–19.

Wool, Charlotte. 2013. "State of the Science on Perinatal Palliative Care. *Journal of Obstetric, Gynecologic, & Neonatal Nursing* 42: 372–82.

Wotta, Laura. 2017. "Liliana's Story." *ChiPPS E-Journal Pediatric Palliative and Hospice Care* 49: 10–11. www.nhpco.org/sites/default/files/public/ChiPPS/ChiPPS_e-journal_Issue-49.pdf (accessed May 16, 2018).

Wrigley, Anthony. 2019. "Hope, Dying and Solidarity." *Ethical Theory and Moral Practice* 22 (1): 187–204.

6 Grief and the Virtue of Compassion

I. Introduction

Beginning in the 1970s, psychologists, obstetricians, and nurses began to document the difficulties of grief following miscarriage, stillbirth, and infant loss.[1] They cataloged a variety of factors that complicate the grief experience, including deficient protocols for addressing the bereavement needs of families. Leon (2008) notes that there was a time when health-care providers

> tried to prevent parents from mourning a stillborn or neonatal death by prohibiting any contact with the dead child, disposing of the body unceremoniously and anonymously, prescribing tranquilizers for the parents to dull any expression of grief, advising them to forget the experience, and often suggesting another pregnancy soon.
>
> (Section 5)

In response to an increased awareness of the grief associated with peri-natal and neonatal death, medical institutions have created new proto-cols for bereavement care including (i) holding and maintaining physical contact with the child's body, (ii) creating keepsakes to memorialize the child's life, (iii) proper and reverent disposal of the child's body, and (iv) mourning rituals following the child's death.[2]

Despite recent advances, there is evidence that healthcare providers and medical institutions compound the experience of grief following an adverse *in utero* diagnosis. Caregivers complicate parents' grief through careless words and behaviors or through an apparent disregard for the family's sorrow.[3] Lang et al. (2011) report that

> more often than not, bereaved parents receive inappropriate or insen-sitive care following a perinatal death, even though there are well accepted standards of care that exists in the theoretical and research literature, as well as among professionals in the field.

(185)

Consider a particularly vivid case.[4] Teresa Streckfuss's son, Benedict, was diagnosed *in utero* with anencephaly, a neural tube defect that results in the absence of a major part of the brain, skull, and scalp. Anencephalic children typically die within a few hours of birth.[5] The individuals who cared for Streckfuss were generally kind but encounters with a thoughtless young doctor compounded her emotional burdens. The physician consistently described the child as nonviable and referred to her as the woman with an 'anencephalic pregnancy.' He failed to acquaint himself with the birth plan—a failure Streckfuss ascribes to arrogance.

Benedict lived for twenty-four hours and thirteen minutes after birth. Unfortunately, the young doctor was on call when Benedict died. Streckfuss narrates her final encounter with him thus:

> He came bursting into our room and listened for Benedict's heartbeat and said, "Okay, that's all fine," before awkwardly leaving us again. Lucky he left. If he hadn't I might have screamed, "THAT'S ALL FINE? THAT'S ALL FINE? GET OUT OF MY ROOM! MY BABY HAS JUST DIED! IT'S NOT ALL FINE! WHAT DO YOU MEAN, THAT'S ALL FINE?" I know what he meant. Our 'non-viable foetus' had died, as expected. He failed to recognise that we had just lost a person, someone we loved. The fact that we knew he would die and accepted this did not make it any less of a loss.
>
> (Reist 2006, 96)

This brief narrative offers a portrait of deficient care for profound grief. To the Streckfuss family, Benedict was a beloved child. His death was not merely the predicted outcome of medical complications; it was the loss of a valued member of their family. His death severed bonds of attachment. It was the cessation of their ability to protect and care for him. It was the disappointment of hopes, wishes, and desires for their child and their family. The physician failed to acknowledge who Benedict was and what he meant to the family; his actions failed to demonstrate an appreciation of the legitimacy of their grief; his callous words and presence signaled an unwillingness to enter into their suffering.

In this chapter, I contrast deficient attitudes and social structures with the compassionate care made possible through the promotion and provision of perinatal hospice. I argue that perinatal hospice manifests the virtue of compassion in its attention to a family's need for consolation. The chapter displays how healthcare providers and institutions can address the family's need for compassionate consolation for their varied griefs. The structure of this chapter is as follows. In Section II, I offer a brief discussion of some general features of grief. Then, I describe some of the unique qualities of grief following a significantly life-limiting antenatal diagnosis. In Section III, I develop an account of the virtue of compassion as an individual virtue—a virtue that takes the needs of the bereaved as a focal object of concern. In Section IV, I show how professional communities and institutions can engage in a common project of consoling families in both their present and anticipatory grief. In Section V, I conclude by describing some of the reforms crucial to ensuring medical institutions and healthcare providers offer fitting consolation for the bereavement needs of affected families.

II. Grief and the Need for Consolation

Grief is one of the most difficult forms of sorrow. In its paradigmatic expressions, it is a profound sadness over the irrevocable loss of a beloved person.[6] But as a general phenomenon, grief is not limited to this form of loss; it concerns the irrevocable loss of important and dearly loved goods either past, present, or future. Grief is rooted in a common human vulnerability: to love is to open oneself to the suffering that results from loss. Grief is a complex emotion issuing in a syndrome of affective, behavioral, conative, and cognitive effects. Over time, grief often gives rise to a range of emotional states including (but not limited to) anger, fear, regret, guilt, and disappointment. It displays itself in both spontaneous acts (e.g., weeping) and structured rituals (e.g., mourning practices). Many of these behaviors have symbolic meaning: they acknowledge the value of the beloved, affirm the legitimacy of felt sadness, and afford opportunities for securing bonds of attachment to the deceased. Grief's effects on perception, attention, and memory are varied. On the one hand, grief can skew, dull, and impair these capacities, causing one to miss or ignore salient features of one's experience. On the other hand, it can focus, heighten, and enhance one's capacity to see, appreciate, and remember significant events and encounters.

Understanding grief requires attending to both its synchronic and diachronic dimensions.[7] As an extended process, grief expresses itself in distinct and varied patterns over time. The bereaved must reorganize their lives around the loss, restructuring their hopes and expectations, their sense of meaning and significance, their sense of normalcy and routine, and, often, the nature of relationships impacted by this loss. Reorienting one's life after loss is a process of negotiating the constant reminders of absence in spaces where there was once a presence.[8] Time does not heal this suffering; it affords ongoing opportunities to navigate life within a context where the beloved is no longer present.[9]

This brief account of some general features of grief provides a framework for considering distinctive dimensions of loss following an adverse *in utero* diagnosis. Consider the range of losses such a diagnosis involves. Families must cope with the loss of (i) a normal pregnancy, (ii) parental or family identity, (iii) relational bonds and attachments, (iv) opportunities for caregiving, (v) hopes, desires, wishes, and dreams for their child and their family, (vi) the child himself, and (vii) the support of caregivers after they leave the hospital.[10] The family experiences these losses in the midst of their attempts to restructure their lives around residual hopes for the child. They grieve an anticipated absence while seeking to honor and take joy in an ongoing presence.

The psychological complexity of this experience alone can challenge a family's capacity to cope with their loss. But this experience is compounded by flawed attitudes and social structures that leave them without comfort or solace in their grief. There is evidence that families encounter these deficiencies within medical institutions. Healthcare providers often fail to acknowledge the child, his value, and his role within the shape and identity of the family. Lang et al. (2011) report encounters between patients and caregivers that minimize "the loss by treating it as a medical event while not recognizing it as the loss of their baby" (191). They add that the "language used by health professionals (e.g., words such as 'spontaneous abortion,' 'miscarriage,' or 'fetal tissue') added to couples' sense of disenfranchisement and contributed to the perception that their loss was insignificant to others" (2011, 191).

Lathrop and VandeVusse (2011a) describe how an adverse diagnosis can alter a mother's sense of identity:

> Mothers' perceptions of themselves as mothers were threatened by the very deaths of their babies. Having a strong bond of attachment and an identity as a mother, in the absence of a living baby, created a sense of unreality and a tendency for mothers to doubt themselves. In addition, many mothers perceived a social bias, that is, an overt or unspoken tendency for others to devalue their babies or their status as mothers. For example, one mother was criticized at her workplace for taking maternity leave, as she had no living infant for whom to care. Others perceived a bias that because their babies were not expected to live very long, they were not expected to form strong attachments and should therefore "get over it" and recover quickly from their losses. Implications that their affected babies were somehow less important than normal babies were particularly upsetting to mothers.
>
> (259)

It is not just mothers who experience the effects of loss as a threat to their identity. Lang et al. (2011) note that fathers report feeling "ignored and unacknowledged as a legitimately grieving parent" (191). Leon (2008) observes,

> Due to not having the visceral affirmation of a woman's motherhood *via* her pregnancy and the social validation of her central reproductive role, fathers may struggle more than their partners with constructing their paternal identity after perinatal loss, especially needing to see the child, possess mementoes [sic] and be recognized as the father.
>
> (Section 4)[11]

Additionally, professional and personal communities sometimes fail to demonstrate an awareness of the legitimacy of their grief. Even if communities acknowledge the loss, they may suggest that it is not as traumatic or difficult as the loss of an older child or an adult. This is, in part, because the early loss of a child has ambivalent status in our culture. Kofod and Brinkman (2017) note, "parental grieving following infant loss requires a constant negotiation of the significance and legitimacy of the loss itself" (530). Negotiations of this kind can signal to the family that the sadness, disappointment, and anger they experience following loss is disproportionate or unwarranted.

Particular institutional structures within medical institutions can compound a family's sense that healthcare providers do not recognize infant death as a real loss. For instance, healthcare providers may discourage parents from seeking birth and death certificates in order to save time and costs associated with filing reports. Malacrida (1999) describes the adverse effects of these practices thus:

> parents themselves often expressed a wish that they had resisted this offer because they had so little in the way of documents and keepsakes to commemorate their children's existence. In our society, certification and paperwork represent legitimacy. Parents of dead babies struggle on every front with a need to have their loss legitimated; the lack of legal documentation represents yet another standard service made unavailable—after all, in what other kind of death would the requisite paperwork be treated as optional?
>
> (514)

Whether intended or not, these structures can disenfranchise a family's grief and complicate their mourning.[12]

Moreover, healthcare providers may add to the burdens of grief by failing to provide a space for meaningful acts of caregiving, memorializing, and securing bonds of attachment with the child. Many families experience perinatal loss in private, without genuine social awareness of the loss and its import—a fact that may lead families to wonder whether their community truly understands its significance. It is uncommon to have funerals or public commemorations that afford recognition of perinatal loss and affirmation for their grief. Additionally, the shortened time for bonding, physical interaction, and embedding the child within their personal community can be an obstacle to expressing grief. Leon (2008) notes, "Grieving demands recollecting the sights, sounds, smells, and touch of the beloved. . . . When the unborn child dies, there is so little to grieve—very limited sensory memories or interactions and, in times past, not even a body to see" (2008, Section 3). Thus, the family has very few experiences to draw upon and to remember as they grieve.

Finally, grief's diachronic dimensions require communities who refuse to place arbitrary time constraints on the family's suffering. The shortness of the child's life may lead some communities to display impatience and discomfort with the family's grief as it extends through time. They may forget important dates and anniversaries. Consequently, parents and family members often commemorate these dates privately, "in keeping with the perceived social norms that undermine the expression of grief surrounding perinatal loss" (Lang et al. 2011, 192).

In spite of the widespread acknowledgement of the difficulties of perinatal loss, a recognition of the importance of bereavement care for affected families, and increased training in grief support, professional and personal communities can adversely impact a family's grief following adverse *in utero* diagnosis. These families need the solace of a community that is sensitive to, appreciative of, and vigilantly concerned for their varied losses. In the next section, I develop an account of the virtue of compassion, an excellence that takes the need for consolation as a focal object of concern.

III. Compassion as an Individual Virtue

The term 'compassion' admits of a wide range of uses across diverse bodies of scholarly literature. Philosophical analyses typically construe compassion as an episodic emotional response to significant suffering.[13] The person who feels compassion is moved to alleviate suffering or to protect a person from its diminishing effects. Recent empirical studies of compassion note that the feeling of compassion also involves a feeling of unease because of the other's suffering and a heightened sensitivity to one's own vulnerability.[14] I do not seek to contest these analyses of compassion; instead, my aim in this section is to offer a profile of compassion that can plausibly be construed as a virtue.

It will be helpful to begin by distinguishing an episodic emotional experience of compassion and the virtue of compassion. The emotion of compassion serves important functions in social life.[15] But there is no guarantee that compassionate emotions are well-tuned. One may experience excessive compassion for minor discomforts or deficient compassion for serious misfortunes. These emotional responses are unmeasured, failing to fit both the degree and severity of the suffering involved. Furthermore, untutored emotions may move a person to act imprudently in the face of serious suffering. Thus, one must carefully distinguish between the basic emotion of compassion and the virtuous expression of compassion. The virtue of compassion gives rise to well-tuned and fitting expressions of compassionate emotions for the sufferer.

As a virtue, compassion is more than the affective expression of caring concern for a person who is suffering. It is a characteristic form of sensitivity to serious suffering such that its perception elicits a pattern of apt affective and behavioral responses toward the sufferer. This is not merely a natural response; it is a deeply-rooted tendency to feel and express affectively attuned and fitting care in the midst of significant sorrow—a regard for the sufferer that displays a sensitivity to his needs, an appreciation of the diminishing effects of suffering, and a commitment to share in his sorrow. This commitment to the project of co-suffering is, perhaps, the chief characteristic of the expression of compassion. Virtuous compassion involves a committed willingness to share in the other's suffering for her sake. It is an excellence that issues in a commitment to take up the other's suffering as one's own—a dispositional willingness to "extend oneself such that the afflicted person can experience her suffering within a relationship of abiding care and felt concern" (Cobb 2018, 52).[16]

In this context, it is important to distinguish between ordinary suffering and the suffering one experiences in feeling compassion for the sufferer. Peter Nilsson (2011) argues that ordinary suffering characteristically places one "in a state or situation that one does not, or would not, want to be in" (127). But the suffering one willingly assumes in expressing virtuous compassion is not properly described as a kind of suffering that one does not or would not want to experience. Although the compassionate person would prefer that suffering did not exist, he willingly assumes suffering as part of what it means to attend properly to the afflicted person. He takes no joy in the need to express compassion, but he gladly wills to share in the project of co-suffering. He does not desire to suffer; rather, he desires to join himself to the sufferer such that the other does not bear the weight of suffering alone. One commits to taking on the other's suffering as one's own in order to help shoulder its burden.

At this point in my analysis, it is instructive to contrast virtuous compassion with some characteristic opposing vices.[17] The first vice one ought to consider is *callousness*, a disposition of hardened disregard for those who are experiencing significant suffering. The callous person may perceive suffering, but it makes no impact on him. The sufferings of others fail to penetrate; they fail to move him. He feels no concern for their sorrow. He is inattentive to their affliction. Given that the sufferings of others cannot get through, he fails to act on the sufferer's behalf. He is characteristically unwilling to share in another's suffering because this suffering does not register as worthy of concern.[18]

Another vice opposing compassion is *aloofness*, an entrenched disposition to withdraw from sharing in the suffering of others. Robert Roberts (2007b) maintains that aloofness characteristically involves a "disinclination to see the commonality between myself and the sufferer I meet, the inclination to dwell on differences between myself and the deficient one—differences that create a distance between him and me" (2007b, 181). Given this kind of distancing, the vice of aloofness involves a dispositional tendency to stand back or move away from the sufferer such that one is not available to share in his suffering. In some forms of aloofness, the person is simply unaffected by the sorrow of another. In other cases, the person may be aloof because of the deep impact such suffering has on him. He may be disposed to withdraw or stand back because the suffering is overwhelming for him.[19] As a result, he will not enter into the sphere of the other's sorrow or commit to engage in the project of co-suffering.[20]

Both callousness and aloofness are vices of deficiency; they stunt a person's capacity for recognizing the diminishing effects of suffering and for enacting bonds vital to addressing others' needs. They also inhibit one's capacity to appreciate and value another's wellbeing as a central aspect of one's moral concern. But there are other flawed expressions of sensitivity to suffering that might be construed as excessive.[21] Lisa Tessman (2005) describes a kind of entrenched anguish characteristic of a person who is "so immersed in the boundless pain of others—and so exhausted with the efforts of ameliorating that pain—that no piece of the self is left free to experience joy or to flourish" (85). This is just one form of excessive sensitivity to the serious sufferings of others—a sensitivity that devastates one's capacity to suffer with and for the sake of others. Anguish is particularly bad because it inhibits a capacity to engage in acts that might enable the sufferer to endure or cope with his sorrow. It encloses a person within a space of excessive concern such that he cannot move toward others and enact bonds vital to enduring suffering. Sufferers may be attuned to the ways their suffering impacts individuals who experience anguish. As a result, they may feel additional burdens because their suffering causes others to experience hardship. They may feel like they need to comfort those who are anguished on their behalf. This effect is another way in which the vice of anguish can be bad for the sufferer.[22]

Another vice in this general domain involves a habitual tendency to become consumed by sorrow on another's behalf. This self-reflexive attention to one's sorrow for the other takes on such salience that it eclipses the afflictions eliciting the concern. Sensitivity to one's own suffering blocks one's capacity to enact a relationship that expresses proper regard and care for the other. What the sufferer needs is someone who will share in his suffering. But the person who is habitually consumed by his own sorrow on the other's behalf fails to engage in this project because of his self-concern.

A number of the vices that oppose compassion also oppose the virtues of hospitality, allocentric hope, and solidarity. This is because there are important interdependencies between this cluster of virtues.[23] Hospitality, allocentric hope, solidarity, and compassion are among those virtues that are rooted in a concern for others' wellbeing and, as such, one and the same action will often manifest each of these virtues. Failures to express one virtue will likely involve failures in the expression of others as well. Thus, in order to focus on the nature of compassion as a distinct virtue, it is important to consider how it is responsive to distinct needs and the distinctive commitments and expressions of compassion especially in relation to these other virtues.

Consider some of the key differences between the virtues of compassion and hospitality. First, the focal concern of compassion is the serious suffering of another person; hospitality focuses on an individual's estrangement from and lack of standing within a particular community. Social exclusion or alienation can be a significant source of suffering because one's lack of standing can make one more susceptible to significant pain and sorrow. But the vulnerabilities rooted in one's status as a stranger can be distinguished from the vulnerabilities one experiences as a sufferer. Compassion focuses on suffering. It disposes a person to take on the project of co-suffering in order to alleviate the sorrow or to enable the sufferer to endure it well. The expression of hospitality may bring a stranger within a space where he can also be the subject of compassion, but its primary focus is on addressing the needs and vulnerabilities of the individual's estrangement.

Another difference between compassion and hospitality is that compassion has a broader scope than hospitality. Hospitality is a virtue that expresses itself in an invitation to the stranger to become a welcome guest within a community. His reception into the community provides a space for belonging, care, and protection. Thus, hospitality characteristically focuses on those outside the community. But one can express virtuous compassion for both those within and those outside of one's community. The need for invitation and welcome is not salient in the context of the suffering of intimates. Furthermore, the expression of virtuous compassion for those outside one's community may not involve the invitation to those individuals into the space and protection of one's community. The relational commitment crucial to compassion can be expressed without inviting the other to join in one's community.[24]

It is also important to distinguish between the virtue of compassion and the virtuous expression of allocentric hope. Here again, we can clarify the differences between these virtues by focusing on the needs that elicit these distinct virtues and their characteristic patterns of expression. The need that elicits compassion is the serious suffering of another person, whereas the focal concern of allocentric hope is the individual who is tempted to hopelessness or despair. There are important connections between the experience of suffering and the temptation to resign all hope. The loss of hope may be a consequence of the experience of serious suffering. The loss of hope can also be a cause of serious suffering. Thus, the compassionate person will take the loss of hope as a serious object of concern in his attempts to address the sufferer's need. The compassionate person may be moved to exercise allocentric hope on behalf of the sufferer as part of the project of co-suffering. Nonetheless, suffering itself does not always tempt one to give up hope. Likewise, the loss of hope may not be a cause of suffering. One's experience of hopelessness and despair may be so complete that one may not feel the absence of hope as something he lacks and ought to lament.[25] These possibilities indicate that the needs that elicit compassion and allocentric hope can be distinguished even if they often co-occur.

One can distinguish between compassion and allocentric hope further in terms of their characteristic expression. Compassion seeks to alleviate or ameliorate suffering through a commitment to suffering with the other. In this way, it involves a distinctive commitment to the other to take on the other's suffering as one's own. Allocentric hope does not always involve this additional commitment to suffer with the other. It expresses itself in an attempt to sustain or inspire another's hope. Often, one will express this kind of hope within the context of one's expression of compassion for the suffering of others. But there is a difference between suffering with another for his sake and hoping on behalf of the other in order that he can maintain or discover hopes worthy of his pursuit.

Finally, it is important to offer some brief remarks concerning the differences between the virtue of compassion and the virtue of solidarity. Both virtues are rooted in an allocentric concern and both involve an affective attunement to the needs of an individual who is suffering. But one can distinguish between the needs that elicit their distinct concern and their distinct behavioral expressions. The need that elicits solidarity is the felt experience of isolation or abandonment. Those who are in these conditions are much more susceptible to suffering; in fact, isolation and abandonment are often a cause of suffering. As I have noted, compassion takes as a focal object of concern the serious suffering of others. Thus, a compassionate person will be moved by the suffering of those who sorrow because of their isolation. And the expression of compassion may lead one to make oneself present to the other so that he knows he is not alone. But one can experience isolation or felt abandonment without experiencing these as a source of suffering. The need for companionship may be present even in those circumstances that do not cause sorrow. Virtuous expressions of solidarity can meet the need for accompaniment independent of the expression of compassion.

Furthermore, one can distinguish these virtues by considering their distinct behavioral expressions. Solidarity is a virtue of joining with and being present to others in a relationship of mutual presence. But being present to a person in this way does not necessarily involve a commitment to share in the other's suffering. So, one may express solidarity without displaying compassion. There is additional commitment internal to the virtue of compassion that moves a person beyond merely being present to the other toward a willing practice of sharing in the other's suffering.

From this extended discussion, one might have a basic sense for compassion as a recognizable form of human excellence. Given the commitments I outlined in the early chapters of this book, however, I need to offer a few words about the ways in which this virtue is crucial to human flourishing. As with previous chapters, I cannot offer a full defense, but I will point to some important considerations that can ground such an account. I begin by considering how the expression of virtuous compassion can benefit those who suffer.

The willingness to share in the sufferings of others can mitigate the afflicted person's experience of suffering. The sufferer may find the weight of sorrow to be less burdensome because he is buoyed up by the commitment of the compassionate person to share in his suffering for his sake. He will see and feel the other's willingness to carry the burden. Additionally, the sufferer may experience a sense of significance in the fact that the compassionate person takes the factors that adversely impact the sufferer's wellbeing as factors that impact his own wellbeing. This commitment communicates to the sufferer that he is worthy of care and concern. Thus, compassionate consolation can impart to the sufferer a clear sense of his value as a person. Serious suffering can challenge a person's sense of worth and the meaning of his life. Expressed compassion can counter false inferences the sufferer may be tempted by concerning his value on account of his suffering.

The virtue of compassion is also a good for the individual who expresses compassion for the sufferer. The exercise of fitting compassion opens one to others and their needs. It makes a person attentive to those in need and, more than this, it draws from him a desire to go to the person in order to join in his suffering. This kind of openness to another—a ready willingness to share in his suffering—is a kind of openness that can create, enact, or deepen bonds vital to human fulfillment. Moreover, one of the consequences of the relational commitment characteristic of the virtue of compassion is a depth in relationship that might not otherwise be possible. There is a deep meaning in sharing in the sufferings of another person. This is a meaning that is discovered only through the expression of fitting compassion through the difficult burden of suffering. The virtuous person will recognize this kind of depth of commitment and attachment as a central value to a well-lived life within a community.

Additionally, compassion involves construing the good of others as a central reason for action. Compassion takes the sufferer and his wellbeing as a focal object of concern. Given the diminishing qualities of suffering, compassion leads the person to desire to suffer with and for the afflicted person in order to address the diminishing effects of suffering. The griefs and pains attending the other's suffering move him to seek out ways to share the weight of the other's sorrow. Furthermore, he sees the suffering of the other as an adverse circumstance he has reason to seek to address. The other's suffering by itself functions as a reason for the virtuous person to act on the other's behalf. The virtuous person is pained by this suffering and, as a result, takes himself to be called to act to address these needs. That the pains and griefs of sufferers are reasons for the person to act is a sign of an expanded vision of what counts as a well-lived human life. If one's reasons for action include the pains and sufferings of others, then one's conception of flourishing extends beyond the limited scope of individual interests. In fact, one has come to think of one's own good as consisting, in part, in how others fare. Cultivating the virtue of compassion enables one to countenance an understanding of one's own good as bound up in the good of others.

Finally, compassion is a virtue essential to the development of communities in which genuine flourishing is possible. Given that we are fragile and dependent beings, we are all vulnerable to serious suffering. We will not be able to flourish unless others are willing to share in our suffering. The failure to cultivate and practice compassion within communities effectively diminishes one's capacity for giving and receiving care for a shared human vulnerability. It is in this context that one can see most clearly the ways in which my analysis of compassion fits with MacIntyre's (1999) general account of the virtues of acknowledged dependence. Cultivating compassion within communities is crucial to fostering the conditions integral to one's own individual flourishing. We are all in a better position to flourish to the extent that individuals in our communities are disposed to participate in the project of co-suffering. This is, in part, because we are better able to tend to tangible needs within these contexts. But it is also because those who possess the virtue of compassion are better able to foster and deepen bonds that are truly conducive to a good and fulfilling human life.

This may be a sufficient analysis of the individual virtue of compassion, but the central aim of this chapter is to argue that perinatal hospice is a common project of care that addresses the family's need for consolation, a focal concern of the virtue of compassion. Therefore, I need to augment this sketch to show how professional communities and their social structures can manifest the virtue of compassion in addressing the bereavement needs of families affected by an adverse *in utero* diagnosis.

IV. Compassion, Common Projects, and Facilitating Structures

I maintain that professional communities or institutions manifest the virtue of compassion through their commitment to a common project of quality bereavement care. The compassionate community is one attuned to the deep sorrow of grief; they recognize the family's needs for acknowledgment, for the affirmation of the legitimacy of their grief, and for an ethos of shared suffering on their behalf. Participation in this common project is not merely an individual task. It is a coordinated effort of a team of people who work together to support each other in meeting the family's needs for consolation. And the institution itself supports caregivers in this compassionate work, recognizing that participating in this kind of bereavement care makes significant demands on their emotional reserves. Institutional support functions as a kind of scaffolding in which healthcare providers are better able to engage in consolatory activities because there is a culture of care for their own emotional needs. It is this structure of nested dependency that enables them to offer quality bereavement care.[26]

Kanov et al.'s (2004) work on organizational compassion offers a helpful framework for thinking about engagement in this kind of common project. On their view, organizational compassion consists in a process of collective noticing, feeling, and responding to the pain of members within an organization. Collective noticing refers to the "collective acknowledgement of pain within a social system such that individuals within the system have a shared appreciation that pain is present" (816). A compassionate organization enables its members to notice pain together because of the ways the organization is structured. The policies, procedures, protocols, and structures foster an ethos that encourages shared sensitivity to and appreciation of the suffering of its members.

Collective feeling is a kind of affect-sharing in which members of an organization feel concern together for the sufferer and "share these feelings more widely with one another" (Kanov et al. 2004, 817). This can occur through either explicit communication or more rudimentary forms of emotion contagion. As with collective noticing, there are social structures that enable or encourage shared affective appreciation of the suffering of members within an organization. For instance, the tone a leader sets through his or her own communication of emotions can contribute to a culture that values sharing in the suffering of others. In organizations with such a culture, "members will be more likely to feel and express empathic concern for those in distress" (Kanov et al. 2004, 818).

Finally, collective responding to suffering involves a concerted effort to act jointly to address the suffering of a member of the organization. Kanov et al. (2004) contend that "an organization's capacity for collective compassionate responding is dependent on its members' heedful interrelating in the face of pain" (820). If there is a culture of consistent and timely acknowledgment of suffering as well as encouragement to respond to suffering throughout levels of the organization, there is a scaffolding for a collective compassionate response.

This framework is helpful for characterizing compassion as an institutional virtue. It is especially valuable for those professional communities whose *raison d'être* concerns the pain and suffering of others in their care. Medical institutions are among those organizations that have this kind of other-regarding focus. Effective policies, practices, and protocols promote social structures of vigilant attention to vulnerable families, affective appreciation and concern for their losses, and coordinated care for their needs. These social structures are central to an ethos of compassionate care. As Leon (2008) notes,

> The bereaved need to know and see that their caregivers care. When caregivers share their sadness, they effectively legitimate grieving for

their patients. This also provides an appropriate channel for caregivers to grieve, which, as long as its intensity does not drown out the loss of the bereaved, should lighten rather than add to the burden of the bereaved.

(Section 4)

But organizational values, practices, policies, and social structures can also inhibit or discourage compassion. Deficient social structures may obstruct a collective response to the sufferings of others. They can facilitate the experience and expression of callous disregard or aloofness toward suffering both within and outside of the organization. In these contexts, institutional structures may undercut healthcare providers in their attempts to support for fitting expressions of grief.

I contend that the provision and promotion of perinatal hospice manifests a different kind of social ethos—one in which families experience compassionate forms of consolation for their grief. Within the supportive spaces of care, they find physicians, nurses, social workers, counselors, chaplains, and others who are committed to offering quality bereavement care. The presence of this professional community does not remove the family's suffering, but it assures them that there is a community willing to share in their sorrow. It communicates that the professional community grasps the gravity of the family's grief and their ongoing need for consolation.

There is perhaps no better way to illustrate this point than to study an exemplary case. At around twenty-five weeks into the pregnancy, the Smith family learned that their unborn child, Matthew, had trisomy 13 and a number of other associated anomalies "including complex congenital heart defect, midline cleft lip, short femurs, pyelectasis, small stomach, and abnormal-appearing feet and genitalia" (Bennett, Dutcher, and Snyders 2011, 74). At the time of diagnosis, the perinatal hospice team met with the family to determine the kind of care they desired to provide. The family opted to provide comfort care at birth, specifically deciding to forgo any extraordinary life-sustaining measures. They indicated to the team their hopes to be able to see and to hold their child, their desire to have the child baptized, and their wish to be in a private room separate from mothers who had given birth to healthy babies. They asked the healthcare providers to call Matthew by his name. After establishing the plan of care, the perinatal hospice team provided a copy of the birth plan to the nursing floor; the team also ensured that a copy of the plan was placed in the mother's medical chart. They reviewed desired care with a resource nurse and the unit manager to ensure effective communication with staff who might be involved in delivering care.

When it came time for delivery, the interdisciplinary team provided the care the Smith family desired. Mr. Smith introduced Matthew to his siblings and grandparents. A member of the perinatal hospice team along with a priest stayed with the family to provide supportive care. After

Matthew's death, the team ensured that the family was able to grieve his loss without interruption. They placed a teardrop card on the door of the room to remind nurses, physicians, and other medical staff to exercise sensitivity in their interactions with the family. Nurses helped the family to create mementos and keepsakes to remember his life. Their care did not stop after the family left the hospital. The nurses involved in their care sent cards to the family three times: one month after birth, during the first holiday after his death, and at the anniversary of his death. Later, the family was invited to attend a commemorative ceremony for families who had experienced perinatal loss.

This brief portrait offers an effective contrast to the deficient care described earlier in this chapter. It illustrates how a professional community may commit to a collective effort of consoling the family in their varied griefs. Bennett, Dutcher, and Snyders (2011) conclude

> This case demonstrates how acknowledgment of family members' grief from the moment of diagnosis through their inpatient stay and beyond provides a venue not only for care delivery, but also for the bereavement process. The advanced care planning developed with the family members identified what was important for them, their child, and their family. It acknowledged the individuality of their child and his needs during birth, his brief life, and his death. It also outlined for the healthcare providers what rituals the family needed to participate in as they experienced their own personal grief.
>
> (75)

In short, within the compassionate care of the perinatal hospice team, the family experienced acknowledgment of their loss, affirmation of the legitimacy of their grief, and the solace of a community attentive to their deep sorrow. In the conclusion, I offer some reflections concerning the steps crucial to ensuring families in need benefit from this kind of care.

V. Conclusion—Fostering a Compassionate Institutional Culture

Creating an institutional culture characterized by compassion may require significant reform in current institutional structures and practices. But one can draw important lessons by considering how structured perinatal hospice programs extend consolation to families in both present and anticipated grief. First, recall that a family's grief is complicated by the lack of acknowledgment of the loss, the value of the child, and the threat to parental and familial identity. As a form of care, perinatal hospice begins with the assumption that the child is a beloved member of the family with whom the family has already established important bonds of loving attachment. Those who meet with the family to construct this plan of care affirm the value of the child by listening to the family and how they want to honor the child's life. They affirm the reality of the parental identity in offering an opportunity to develop a plan of care that enables and facilitates parental acts of caregiving. The perinatal hospice team creates an ethos that affords multiple opportunities for families to engage in memory-making and deepening bonds of attachment. For instance, they can provide additional opportunities to hear the child's heartbeat and to receive ultrasound pictures.

Second, when the child is born, the perinatal hospice team can provide opportunities for the family to engage in acts of care. The family can hold, bathe, dress, and feed the child; they can participate in significant rituals such as baptism. The family can introduce the child to extended family and friends, thus ensuring that his presence is embedded within their personal community. This process is a key dimension of social acknowledgment; it enables the community to recognize, receive, and appreciate the child as a member of the community itself. Caregivers and professional photographers can help the family by creating and providing meaningful keepsakes. All of these activities foster an ethos of acknowledgment concerning the family's loss, affirmation of the legitimacy of grief, and support for proper mourning.

Third, the team can sensitively prepare the family for the child's death. This kind of anticipatory guidance can help the family to make the most of the short time while diminishing the chances that they will experience trauma during the dying process. At the death of the child, they can support the family in final acts of caregiving, including the ultimate act of entrusting the body into the hands of healthcare providers. The medical team can facilitate proper planning for rituals following death, including addressing the disposition of the child's body and preparation for funeral and burial. These practices can help the family come to terms with the finality of death. Simultaneously, the practices affirm for the family that they have done everything they could to provide the best kind of care possible for the child.

Fourth, the perinatal hospice team can continue to provide for the family after death by reaching out to them at significant intervals after death with notes and remembrances. These activities acknowledge the diachronic experience of grief following loss. The team communicates their recognition that the family needs to remain bonded with the child even as they orient their lives around this loss. As Romesberg (2004) notes,

> When an infant dies in the NICU, the family leaves behind the support systems and relationships that they established in the hospital. This abrupt end to contact may feel like abandonment. In addition, they may return home to find family and friends who are not supportive and understanding of their experience. Grief follow-up programs enable established relationships to continue after the death,

which allows time for grief and sharing of feelings, and therefore facilitates the parents' ability to move successfully through the stages of grief.

(167–168)[27]

As Romesberg emphasizes, social support networks for bereaved families are crucial in the provision of compassionate consolation for the family. While symbolic acts of writing notes or remembrances may be helpful, the personal connections established in grief support groups are much more likely to provide the interpersonal consolation characteristic of the virtue of compassion.

Sadly, many families do not experience these kinds of consolation within medical institutions or their personal communities. One factor that may contribute to this unmet need is a concern about the emotional burdens of participating in the suffering of these families. Compassion can make significant demands on caregivers' emotional reserves—demands that threaten to overwhelm the healthcare provider's capacity to offer effective care.[28] As a result, physicians, nurses, and other caregivers may be tempted to detach or distance themselves from affected families. This is especially the case if a medical institution promotes a culture in which only a few individuals (predominantly nurses) must bear most of the weight of bereavement care.

Another barrier to compassionate consolation may be rooted in protocols and policies of medical institutions. As Fotaki (2015) notes,

> organisational cultures, policies and politics might exert a damaging influence on caring values. Shift towards impersonal surveillance systems coupled with cost savings measures imposed by those who are distanced from the reality of care militates against developing compassionate caring institutions.

(201)

These structures encode engagement between and among healthcare providers and patients. Some structures may undercut any efforts to expand medical practice to the consoling efforts characteristic of fitting bereavement care. Within these structures, physicians and nurses may find it difficult to engage in consolatory activities.

Given these barriers, what needs to occur to foster more compassionate institutions for families who have received an adverse *in utero* diagnosis? First, one must address the culture within medical institutions that inhibits consolatory activity. Although doctors cannot alleviate the sorrow of grief, they have a range of skills and capacities that can facilitate acknowledgment of loss, validation of grief, and support for the expressions of mourning. Arguably, consolation is a constituent part of medical care.[29] Medicine is not merely a technique for curing illness and disease; it is an allocentric practice oriented toward healing and wholeness. In contexts where health and function cannot be restored, practitioners express other-regarding concern by sharing in the experience of suffering with their patients. This care creates a trustworthy relational foundation for those who suffer; they know that the healthcare providers are committed to suffering with them and on their behalf. Especially in the moments following death, affective engagement with families is itself a great comfort. Grieving with the family in the intimate moments following death is both natural and fitting given the loss. Furthermore, the family who sees healthcare providers grieving with them may find solace in the expressed sadness on their behalf. Expressed affective attunement to the family in their loss is a sign of acknowledgment, affirmation, and apt mourning.

The second step to removing barriers to compassionate care involves addressing the concern about emotional distress and burnout. Here it is worth noting that the evidence concerning the role of compassion fatigue in emotional burnout does not, at present, justify the claim that compassionate engagement with patients inevitably leads to burnout. In fact, there is some evidence that expressed compassion may be vital to avoiding emotional burnout in healthcare workers. As Michael Spezio (2015) notes, recent research "with real-world compassionate action shows that emotional increases in emotional resonance with another person's pain associated with *lower* emotional exhaustion on the job" (35).[30] Leon (2008) writes,

> Early work exploring the reactions of medical caregivers to perinatal loss focused on their tendency to resort to psychological defenses to protect themselves against the range of intense feelings resulting from these losses. Essentially, by avoiding as much contact as possible with the bereaved, by not thinking about or remembering those losses, by intellectualizing or rationalizing their reactions, and even, sometimes, by blaming the bereaved, medical caregivers could successfully still their own feelings of sadness, guilt, and inadequacy. This temporary relief of their own distress was bought, however, at the high price of failing to meaningfully engage with their bereaved patients, and effective coping was blocked as a result of their warded-off feelings.
>
> (Section 4)

Thus, there is reason to question the view that adopting a guarded emotional stance in the context of grief is best for healthcare providers.

Nonetheless, given the emotional demands of the virtue of compassion, healthcare providers must be attentive to the possibility of emotional fatigue; personal distress over the grief of an affected family may compromise the ability to offer fitting care. Medical institutions can demonstrate virtuous concern for this possibility by ensuring that physicians and nurses tasked with caring for these families receive sufficient support for their own sorrow.[31] Hospital administrators need to ensure that they are attentive to and concerned for the grief physicians and nurses experience as they commit to the difficult work of consolation. In this way, institutions can support and scaffold the ongoing work of caregivers as they address the suffering of their patients. Emotional burnout may be less likely within institutions that prioritize and promote an ethos of compassion throughout the organization.

By promoting and providing perinatal hospice, medical institutions respond to needs that are at the heart of the virtue of compassion. They create structures that can provide fitting care for the deep needs associated with grief. Families who receive an adverse *in utero* diagnosis experience significant loss. They need personal and professional communities to provide a supportive ethos for fitting expressions of grief. Professional communities who engage in these activities together participate in a common project that extends compassionate consolation to the family. When these activities take place within a culture of encouragement for consolatory work, there are structures of nested dependency that provide a scaffolding of support crucial for engaging compassionately with those in need. Professional communities that promote and provide perinatal hospice display virtue in response to the bereavement needs of families following an adverse antenatal diagnosis. Shared commitment to and engagement in quality bereavement care is a good common project. Structured programs in perinatal hospice manifest the virtue of compassion through this sensitive and attuned work of consolation.

Notes

1 See Leon (2008) for discussion of this historical context.
2 For extensive discussion, see Gold, Dalton, and Schwenk (2007).
3 For similar results, see Gold (2007).
4 See Reist (2006) for the full narrative.
5 Nonetheless, there are children who defy the odds. Jaquier, Klein, and Boltshauser (2006) studied 211 pregnancies in which there was a diagnosis of anencephaly: of the 153 pregnancies in which the child was born alive, six children lived longer than six days; one child lived for twenty-eight days after birth. Dickman, Fletke, and Redfern (2016) report on the longest known survivor with anencephaly, a child who lived twenty-eight months after birth.
6 None of the general claims about the experience of grief in this section should be taken to imply that one can fully comprehend the intensely personal nature of grief. In what follows, I have benefitted from the following reflections on grief: Cholbi (2013, 2017); Goldie (2011); Gustafson (1989); Jakoby (2012); Kristjánsson (2015); and Ratcliffe (2017).
7 For discussion, see, especially, Goldie (2011) and Cholbi (2013).
8 See, especially, Ratcliffe (2017).
9 See Jakoby (2012).
10 For discussion of a range of studies documenting these kinds of losses and the vital role of caregivers in addressing perinatal bereavement, see Fenstermacher and Hupcey (2013); Foster, Kain, and Patterson (2016); Furman (1978); Gandino et al. (2017); Gold (2007); Gold, Dalton, and Schwenk (2007); Kersting

and Wagner (2012); Kobler and Limbo (2011) Kofod and Brinkmann (2017); Lathrop and VandeVusse (2011a, 2011b); Lang et al. (2011); Leon (2008); Limbo and Kobler (2010); Limbo and Lathrop (2014); Limbo, Lathrop, and Heustis (2015); Locock, Crawford, and Crawford (2005); Malacrida (1999); McCreight (2004); Moyle-Wright and Hogan (2008); Romesberg (2004); Roose and Blanford (2011); Rosenbaum, Smith, and Zollfrank (2011); Williams et al. (2008); and Wool and Catlin (2018).

11 I noted early in this book that common experiences and needs can impact individuals in distinct ways. The varied effects of loss on parents is one instance of this kind; their unique experiences of loss and grief will affect them differently even if both need consolation for their loss. Likewise, a sibling's experience of loss and grief will vary from the parents. Thus, virtuous consolation must be attentive to the distinct nature of these common needs.

12 On disenfranchised grief, see Attig (2004); Corr (1999); Doka (1989, 2002). On complicated mourning, see Kersting and Wagner (2012); Rando (1993).

13 Some scholars employ the terms 'sympathy' and 'compassion' interchangeably. But others distinguish between sympathy, which they take to be a fitting response for trivial forms of suffering or personal discomfort, and compassion, which they construe as a proper response to *serious* suffering. For further discussion of sympathy, see Ben-Ze'ev (2000); Darwall (1998); Kristjánsson (2014); and Snow (1991, 2013).

14 See Goetz, Keltner, and Simon-Thomas (2010); Sinclair et al. (2016, 2018); and Strauss et al. (2016). Poore (2018) denies the claim that compassion involves this kind of heightened sensitivity.

15 For a range of contemporary philosophical discussions of compassion, see Blum (1980); Caouette and Price (2018); Crisp (2008); Goldie (2002); Nilsson (2011); Nussbaum (1996, 2001, 2003); Roberts (2007a, 2007b, 2016); and Snow (1991).

16 To underscore this relational commitment characteristic of virtuous compassion, it is helpful to contrast it with other forms of other-regarding affective concern. In endnote 13, I noted some potential differences between compassion and sympathy. One can add to these that the expression of sympathy does not involve any commitment to share in another's suffering. One can also distinguish between compassion and empathy. Empathy is an other-oriented and other-focused perspective-taking that enables one to experience emotions similar in kind to the affected person and to understand, in part, how he feels. There are two primary differences between compassion and empathy. First, one can express empathic regard for a sufferer without any commitment to share in his suffering. Second, although empathy may involve a desire to alleviate another person's suffering, it does not necessarily issue in this kind of concern. Through empathic perspective-taking, a cruel person may experience enjoyment in others' suffering. For helpful philosophical discussions of empathy, see Ben-Ze'ev (2000); Coplan (2011); Coplan and Goldie (2011); Darwall (1998, 2011); Kristjánsson (2014); Miller (2011, 2015); Snow (2000); and Trivigno (2014). Empirical studies of compassion also draw distinctions between empathy and compassion. See, in particular, Strauss et al. (2016, 18–19). Finally, one can distinguish compassion and pity. Pity often expresses itself in a kind of distancing from the sufferer. At times, this withdrawal displays itself in contempt for the pitiable state of the sufferer. Compassion, on the other hand, disposes the person to identify with the vulnerability of the sufferer as a common form of human frailty. It disposes the person to move toward the sufferer such that he can be with him and share in his sorrow. For further discussions of pity, see Ben-Ze'ev (2000); Callan (1988); Kristjánsson (2014); and Nuyen (1999). Kristjánsson (2014) argues that pity may play an important role in the cultivation of virtue.

17 As in earlier chapters, however, I think it is important to distinguish between a failure to manifest virtue and the expression of vice. One may fail to express proper compassion without being vicious. Given the distinctive affective, behavioral, and cognitive dimensions of the virtue of compassion, there are many ways one may miss the mark without possessing one of the specific vices I profile.

18 There are a number of concerns that may feed callousness toward a sufferer, including apathy, fear of the potential discomfort of opening oneself to suffering on another's behalf, or a general contentment with one's comfort. As Miner (2015) notes, "Failure to feel compassion is not caused by some obvious, easily identified vice. It is generated by a range of factors that render a person unable to recognise her real union with other human beings" (78).

19 I would like to thank Gregory Poore for helping me to see the need to state this point with greater care.

20 It is important to note that the vice of aloofness involves an emotional and relational distancing that is also incompatible with the virtue of solidarity.

21 Roger Crisp (2008), for instance, construes a misdirected kind of compassion for a disabled person because of his physical appearance as an expression of excessive or "inappropriate pity" (242).

22 I'm grateful to Gregory Poore for drawing my attention to this possibility.

23 See Gulliford and Roberts (2018) for discussion of the clustering of allocentric virtues.

24 Another difference between these virtues concerns their respective relationships with the virtue of justice. Although hospitality is often rooted in a concern for the wellbeing of the stranger, it is closely linked with what we owe to others in virtue of their humanity. The failure to be hospitable to the stranger is also a failure to exercise justice. The connection between compassion and justice is not as clear. Some analyses of compassion maintain that compassion for the serious suffering resulting from a person's moral flaws or culpable failings is misplaced. Compassion is fittingly expressed only if it targets individuals who deserve compassionate regard. If the individual sufferers because of culpable failings, he does not deserve compassionate regard and expressed compassion is inapt. Thus, a failure to express compassion is not always a failure of justice. But not all analyses maintain this connection between compassion and justice. Thus, the relationship between compassion and justice can be distinguished from the connections between hospitality and justice. See Roberts (2007a) and (2016) for further discussion of this point.

25 For further discussion, see Ratcliffe (2013).

26 On nested dependence, see Kittay (1999, 2011).

27 See Calhoun (2010) for further discussion of postpartum grief support within perinatal hospice programs.

28 For recent discussion, see Barr (2017).

29 For an articulation of this view, see Norberg, Bergsten, and Lundman (2001).

30 Spezio cites Tei et al. (2014) in support of this claim.

31 For discussion of the way institutions can more effectively address the emotional needs of healthcare providers in these contexts, see Gandino et al. (2017).

References

Attig, Thomas. 2004. "Disenfranchised Grief Revisited: Discounting Hope and Love." *OMEGA-Journal of Death and Dying* 49 (3): 197–215.

Barr, Peter. 2017. "Compassion Fatigue and Compassion Satisfaction in Neonatal Intensive Care Unit Nurses: Relationships with Work Stress and Perceived social Support." *Traumatology* 23 (2): 214–22.

Bennett, Joann, Janet Dutcher, and Michele Snyders. 2011. "Embrace: Addressing Anticipatory Grief and Bereavement in the Perinatal Population: A Palliative Care Case Study." *The Journal of Perinatal & Neonatal Nursing* 25 (1): 72–6.

Ben-Ze'ev, Aaron. 2000. *The Subtlety of Emotions*. Cambridge, MA: MIT Press.

Blum, Lawrence. 1980. "Compassion." In *Explaining Emotions*, edited by Amelia Rorty, 507–18. Berkeley: University of California Press.

Calhoun, Byron D. 2010. "Perinatal Hospice: Compassionate and Comprehensive Care for Families with Lethal Prenatal Diagnosis." *The Linacre Quarterly* 77 (2): 147–56.

Callan, Eamonn. 1988. "The Moral Status of Pity." *Canadian Journal of Philosophy* 18 (1): 1–12.

Caouette, Justin and Carolyn Price. 2018. *The Moral Psychology of Compassion*. London and New York: Rowman & Littlefield.

Cholbi, Michael. 2013. "Grief." *International Encyclopedia of Ethics*: 1–7.

Cholbi, Michael. 2017. "Grief's Rationality, Backward and Forward." *Philosophy and Phenomenological Research* 94 (2): 255–72.

Cobb, Aaron D. 2018. "Compassion and Consolation." In *The Moral Psychology of Compassion*, edited by Justin Caouette and Carolyn Price, 49–60. London and New York: Rowman & Littlefield.

Coplan, Amy and Peter Goldie. 2011. *Empathy: Philosophical and Psychological Perspectives*. Oxford: Oxford University Press.

Coplan, Amy. 2011. "Will the Real Empathy Please Stand Up? A Case for Narrow Conceptualization." *Southern Journal of Philosophy* 49 (s1): 40–65.

Corr, Charles A. 1999. "Enhancing the Concept of Disenfranchised Grief." *OMEGA-Journal of Death and Dying* 38 (1): 1–20.

Crisp, Roger. 2008. "Compassion and Beyond." *Ethical Theory and Moral Practice* 11 (3): 233–46.

Darwall, Stephen. 1998. "Empathy, Sympathy, Care." *Philosophical Studies* 89 (2–3): 261–82.

Darwall, Stephen. 2011. "Being With." *Southern Journal of Philosophy* 49 (s1): 4–24.

Dickman, Holly, Kyle Fletke, and Roberta E. Redfern. 2016. "Prolonged Unassisted Survival in an Infant with Anencephaly." *BMJ Case Reports*.

Doka, Kenneth J. 1989. "Disenfranchised Grief." In *Disenfranchised Grief: Recognizing Hidden Sorrow*, edited by Kenneth J. Doka, 1–13. Lexington, MA: Lexington Press.

Doka, Kenneth J. 2002. *Disenfranchised Grief: New Directions, Challenges and Strategies for Practice*. Champaign, IL: Research Press.

Fenstermacher, Kimberly and Judith E. Hupcey. 2013. "Perinatal Bereavement: A Principle-based Concept Analysis." *Journal of Advanced Nursing* 69 (11): 2389–400.

Foster, Jann, Victoria Kain, and Tiffany Patterson. 2016. "Parents' and Families' Experiences of Palliative and End-of-Life Neonatal Care in Neonatal Settings: A Systematic Review Protocol." *JBI Database of Systematic Reviews and Implementation Reports* 14 (11): 99–105.

Fotaki, Marianna. 2015. "Why and How is Compassion Necessary to Provide Good Quality Healthcare?" *International Journal of Health Policy and Management* 4 (4): 199–201.

Furman, Ema. 1978. "The Death of the Newborn: Care of the Parents." *Birth* 5 (4): 214–18.

Gandino, Gabriella, Antonella Bernaudo, Giulia Di Fini, Ilaria Vanni, and Fabio Veglia. 2017. "Healthcare Professionals' Experiences of Perinatal Loss: A Systematic Review." *Journal of Health Psychology* 1359105317705981: 1–14.

Goetz, Jennifer L., Dacher Keltner, and Emiliana Simon-Thomas. 2010. "Compassion: An Evolutionary Analysis and Empirical Review." *Psychological Bulletin* 136 (3): 351–74.

Gold, Katherine J. 2007. "Navigating Care after a Baby Dies: A Systematic Review of Parent Experiences with Health Providers." *Journal of Perinatology* 27 (4): 230–7.

Gold, Katherine J., Vanessa K. Dalton, and Thomas L. Schwenk. 2007. "Hospital Care for Parents After Perinatal Death." *Obstetrics & Gynecology* 109 (5): 1156–66.

Goldie, Peter. 2002. "Compassion: A Natural, Moral Emotion." In *Die Moralität der Gefühle*, edited by Verena Mayer & Sabine A. Döring, 199–212. Berlin: De Gruyter.

Goldie, Peter. 2011. "Grief: A Narrative Account." *Ratio* 24 (2): 119–37.

Gulliford, Liz and Robert C. Roberts. 2018. "Exploring the 'Unity' of the Virtues: The Case of an Allocentric Quintet." *Theory & Psychology* 28 (2): 208–26.

Gustafson, Donald. 1989. "Grief." *Noûs* 23 (4): 457–79.

Jakoby, Nina R. 2012. "Grief as a Social Emotion: Theoretical Perspectives." *Death studies* 36 (8): 679–711.

Jaquier, Minoka, Andrea Klein, and Eugen Boltshauser. 2006. "Spontaneous Pregnancy Outcome after Prenatal Diagnosis of Anencephaly." *BJOG: An International Journal of Obstetrics & Gynaecology* 113 (8): 951–3.

Kanov, Jason M., Sally Maitlis, Monica C. Worline, Jane E. Dutton, Peter J. Frost, and Jacoba M. Lilius. 2004. "Compassion in Organizational Life." *American Behavioral Scientist* 47 (6): 808–27.

Kersting, Anette and Birgit Wagner. 2012. "Complicated Grief after Perinatal Loss." *Dialogues in Clinical Neuroscience* 14 (2): 187–94.

Kittay, Eva Feder. 1999. *Love's Labor: Essays on Women, Equality and Dependency*. London: Routledge.

Kittay, Eva Feder. 2011. "The Ethics of Care, Dependence, and Disability." *Ratio Juris* 24 (1): 49–58.

Kobler, Kathie and Rana Limbo. 2011. "Making a Case: Creating a Perinatal Palliative Care Service Using a Perinatal Bereavement Program Model." *The Journal of Perinatal & Neonatal Nursing* 25 (1): 32–41.

Kofod, Ester Holte and Svend Brinkmann. 2017. "Grief as a Normative Phenomenon: The Diffuse and Ambivalent Normativity of Infant Loss and Parental Grieving in Contemporary Western Culture." *Culture & Psychology* 23 (4): 519–33.

Kristjánsson, Kristján. 2014. "Pity: A Mitigated Defence." *Canadian Journal of Philosophy* 44 (3–4): 343–64.

Kristjánsson, Kristján. 2015. "Grief: An Aristotelian Justification of an Emotional Virtue." *Res Philosophica* 92 (4): 805–28.

Lang, Ariella, Andrea R. Fleiszer, Fabie Duhamel, Wendy Sword, Kathleen R. Gilbert, and Serena Corsni-Munt. 2011. "Perinatal Loss and Parental Grief: The Challenge of Ambiguity and Disenfranchised Grief." *OMEGA-Journal of Death and Dying* 63 (1): 183–96.

Lathrop, Anthony and Leona VandeVusse. 2011a. "Affirming Motherhood: Validation and Invalidation in Women's Perinatal Hospice Narratives." *Birth* 38 (3): 256–65.

Lathrop, Anthony and Leona VandeVusse. 2011b. "Continuity and Change in Mothers' Narratives of Perinatal Hospice." *The Journal of Perinatal & Neonatal Nursing* 25 (1): 21–31.

Leon, Irving G. 2008. "Helping Families Cope with Perinatal Loss." *The Global Library of Women's Medicine.* www.glowm.com/section_view/item/417/recordset/18975/value/417 (accessed May 10, 2018).

Limbo, Rana and Anthony Lathrop. 2014. "Caregiving in Mothers' Narratives of Perinatal Hospice." *Illness, Crisis & Loss* 22 (1): 43–65.

Limbo, Rana and Kathie Kobler. 2010. "The Tie That Binds: Relationships in Perinatal Bereavement." *MCN: The American Journal of Maternal/Child Nursing* 35 (6): 316–21.

Limbo, Rana K., Anthony Lathrop, and Jane Heustis. 2015. "Caregiving as a Theoretical Framework in Perinatal Palliative Care." In *Perinatal and Pediatric Bereavement in Nursing and Other Health Professions,* edited by Beth Perry Black, Patricia Moyle Wright, and Rana Limbo, 33–54. New York: Springer Publishing.

Locock, Louise, Jane Crawford, and Jon Crawford. 2005. "The Parents' Journey: Continuing a Pregnancy after a Diagnosis of Patau's Syndrome." *BMJ: British Medical Journal* 331 (7526): 1186–9.

MacIntyre, Alasdair C. 1999. *Dependent Rational Animals: Why Human Beings Need the Virtues.* Chicago, IL: Open Court.

Malacrida, Claudia. 1999. "Complicating Mourning: The Social Economy of Perinatal Death." *Qualitative Health Research* 9 (4): 504–19.

McCreight, Bernadette Susan. 2004. "A Grief Ignored: Narratives of Pregnancy Loss from a Male Perspective." *Sociology of Health & Illness* 26 (3): 326–50.

Miller, Christian. 2011. "Defining Empathy: Thoughts on Coplan's Approach." *Southern Journal of Philosophy* 49 (s1): 66–72.

Miller, Christian. 2015. "Empathy as the Only Hope for the Virtue of Compassion and as Support for a Limited Unity of the Virtues." *Philosophy, Theology, and the Sciences* 2 (1): 89–113.

Miner, Robert C. 2015. "The Difficulties of Mercy: Reading Thomas Aquinas on Misericordia." *Studies in Christian Ethics* 28 (1): 70–85.

Moyle-Wright, Patricia and Nancy S. Hogan. 2008. "Grief Theories and Models: Applications to Hospice Nursing Practice." *Journal of Hospice & Palliative Nursing* 10 (6): 350–6.

Nilsson, Peter. 2011. "On the Suffering of Compassion." *Philosophia* 39 (1): 125–44.

Norberg, Astrid, Monica Bergsten, and Berit Lundman. 2001. "A Model of Consolation." *Nursing Ethics* 8 (6): 544–53.

Nussbaum, Martha C. 2001. *Upheavals of Thought: The Intelligence of Emotions.* Cambridge: Cambridge University Press.

Nussbaum, Martha C. 2003. "Compassion & Terror." *Daedalus* 132 (1): 10–26.

Nussbaum, Martha. 1996. "Compassion: The Basic Social Emotion." *Social Philosophy and Policy* 13 (1): 27–58.

Nuyen, A.T. 1999. "Pity." *Southern Journal of Philosophy* 37 (1): 77–87.

Poore, Gregory S. 2018. "The Role of Similar Vulnerability in Aristotle's Account of Compassion." *Ancient Philosophy* 38 (2): 347–55.

Rando, Therese A. 1993. *Treatment of Complicated Mourning.* Champaign, IL: Research Press.

Ratcliffe, Matthew. 2013. "What is it to Lose Hope?" *Phenomenology and the Cognitive Sciences* 12 (4): 597–614.

Ratcliffe, Matthew. 2017. "Grief and the Unity of Emotion." *Midwest Studies in Philosophy* 41 (1): 154–74.

Reist, Melinda Tankard. 2006. *Defiant Birth: Women Who Resist Medical Eugenics*. North Melbourne: Spinifex Press.

Roberts, Robert C. 2007a. "Compassion as an Emotion and as a Virtue." In *Mitleid: Konkretionen Eines Strittigen Konzepts*, edited by Ingolf U. Dalferth, 119–37. Tübingen: Mohr Siebeck.

Roberts, Robert C. 2007b. *Spiritual Emotions: A Psychology of Christian Virtues*. Grand Rapids, MI: Wm. B. Eerdmans Publishing Co.

Roberts, Robert C. 2016. "Emotions in the Christian Tradition," *The Stanford Encyclopedia of Philosophy*, edited by Edward N. Zalta. https://plato.stanford.edu/archives/win2016/entries/emotion-Christian-tradition (accessed May 10, 2018).

Romesberg, Tricia L. 2004. "Understanding Grief: A Component of Neonatal Palliative Care." *Journal of Hospice & Palliative Nursing* 6 (3): 161–70.

Roose, Rosmarie E. and Cathy R. Blanford. 2011. "Perinatal Grief and Support Spans the Generations: Parents' and Grandparents' Evaluations of an Intergenerational Perinatal Bereavement Program." *The Journal of Perinatal & Neonatal Nursing* 25 (1): 77–85.

Rosenbaum, Joan L., Joan Renaud Smith, and Reverend Zollfrank. 2011. "Neonatal End-of-Life Spiritual Support Care." *The Journal of Perinatal & Neonatal Nursing* 25 (1): 61–9.

Sinclair, Shane, Jill M. Norris, Shelagh J. McConnell, Harvey Max Chochinov, Thomas F. Hack, Neil A. Hagen, Susan McClement, and Shelley Raffin Bouchal. 2016. "Compassion: A Scoping Review of the Healthcare Literature." *BMC Palliative Care* 15 (1): 6–20.

Sinclair, Shane, Thomas F. Hack, Shelley Raffin-Bouchal, Susan McClement, Kelli Stajduhar, Pavneet Singh, Neil A. Hagen, Aynharan Sinnarajah, and Harvey Max Chochinov. 2018. "What are Healthcare Providers' Understandings and Experiences of Compassion? The Healthcare Compassion Model: A Grounded Theory Study of Healthcare Providers in Canada." *BMJ Open* 8 (3): p.e019701.

Snow, Nancy E. 1991. "Compassion." *American Philosophical Quarterly* 28 (3): 195–205.

Snow, Nancy E. 2000. "Empathy." *American Philosophical Quarterly* 37 (1): 65–78.

Snow, Nancy E. 2013. "Sympathy." In *The International Encyclopedia of Ethics*, edited by Hugh LaFollette, 5101–8. Chichester: Wiley-Blackwell.

Spezio, Michael. 2015. "Embodied Cognition and Loving Character Empathy and Character in Moral Formation." *Philosophy, Theology and the Sciences* 2 (1): 25–40.

Strauss, Clara, Billie Lever Taylor, Jenny Gu, Willem Kuyken, Ruth Baer, Fergal Jones, and Kate Cavanagh. 2016. "What is Compassion and How Can We Measure It? A Review of Definitions and Measures." *Clinical Psychology Review* 47: 15–27.

Tei, Shisei, Carl Becker, Ryousaku Kawada, Junya Fujino, Kathryn F. Jankowski, Gau Sugihara, Toshiya Murai, and Hidehiko Takahashi. 2014. "Can We Predict Burnout Severity from Empathy-related Brain Activity?" *Translational Psychiatry* 4 (6): e393–97.

Tessman, Lisa. 2005. *Burdened Virtues: Virtue Ethics for Liberatory Struggles.* Oxford: Oxford University Press.

Trivigno, Franco V. 2014. "Empathic Concern and the Pursuit of Virtue." In *The Philosophy and Psychology of Character and Happiness*, edited by Nancy E. Snow and Franco V. Trivigno, 113–32. London: Routledge.

Williams, Constance, David Munson, John Zupancic, and Haresh Kirpalani. 2008. "Supporting Bereaved Parents: Practical Steps in Providing Compassionate Perinatal and Neonatal End-of-life Care—A North American Perspective." *Seminars in Fetal and Neonatal Medicine* 13 (5): 335–40.

Wool, Charlotte and Anita Catlin. 2018. "Perinatal Bereavement and Palliative Care Offered Throughout the Healthcare System." *Annals of Palliative Medicine* 8 (1): S22–S29.

7 Virtuous Projects of Social, Structural, and Institutional Reform

I. Introduction

This book has been an extended essay in applied virtue ethics. I sketched profiles of four virtues, each of which takes human vulnerability and need as a focal object of concern: hospitality, hope, solidarity, and compassion.[1] Each of these virtues involves a characteristic sensitivity to common human vulnerabilities; all of them issue in patterns of movement outward from the self toward those in need.[2] While these virtues are often characterized as excellences of individual persons, I suggested that one can ascribe these virtues to communities and institutions in virtue of their shared commitment to and participation in a good common project.[3] The application of this framework is straightforward: perinatal hospice teams are engaged in a good common project of addressing the needs and vulnerabilities of families who have received an adverse *in utero* diagnosis. To the extent that this collective effort addresses the family's needs for welcome, meaning, accompaniment, and consolation, commitment to this project manifests the virtues of hospitality, hope, solidarity, and compassion.

In each chapter, I highlighted structured programs of care to show how they respond with sensitivity and attunement to the unique dimensions of the experience of continuing a pregnancy following antenatal diagnosis of a significantly life-limiting condition. These programs coordinate and integrate the tasks of an interdisciplinary team, often working across institutional settings, such that they can provide seamless care. Attending to these exemplary programs draws attention to the deficiencies of common practices and social structures within many contemporary care settings. As models, they provide guidance for the reformation of practices and social structures that fail to express virtue or, worse, manifest vice.

One important implication of my account is that individual healthcare providers, professional communities, and medical institutions ought to pursue these reforms. Fulfilling these tasks involves a range of activities including the following: ensuring access to care for families in need; promoting awareness of these forms of care within medical institutions, among healthcare providers, and within the broader population; and addressing or rectifying cultures and practices of care that inhibit awareness of, access to, or delivery of care. Individual healthcare providers are already working diligently to address the needs of affected families. But these efforts alone cannot remedy the structural barriers many confront as they seek to secure care. These families need more than the expression of individual virtue; social and structural deficiencies require social and structural remedies. The primary aim of this chapter is to identify and address some of the chief barriers to reform within professional communities and medical institutions. But before I can engage in these tasks, I need to highlight the value of the *virtue-based* defense I have developed in this work.

The structure of this chapter is as follows. In Section II, I contrast the *virtue-based* defense of perinatal hospice with alternative views, emphasizing some of the distinctive dimensions of my account. In Section III, I identify and describe barriers that may hinder the reforms crucial to the promotion and provision of these forms of care. Finally, in Section IV, I conclude with an extended reflection on the goods enacted through perinatal hospice. Drawing on my family's experience as beneficiaries of perinatal hospice, I point to these goods both as a foundation justifying the pursuit of structural reform and a reason to hope that such reforms are realizable.

II. The Distinctive Value of a Virtue-Based Defense of Perinatal Hospice

In Chapter 1, I distinguished three basic approaches to the ethics of perinatal hospice.[4] According to the *moral status* defense, perinatal hospice is valuable because it respects the inherent worth and dignity of the unborn child. Typically, this defense is rooted in a theological account of human dignity according to which the unborn child is a person created in the image of God. The *reproductive autonomy* defense maintains that perinatal hospice is valuable because it respects the choices of families who desire to continue a pregnancy. The *supportive care* defense maintains that perinatal hospice is valuable because it aligns quality medical care with family commitments and values.

Each of these accounts has important strengths, but the criticisms I offered in Chapter 1 suggest that they are limited and need to be supplemented by appeals to other important goods or values. I have not offered extended criticism of these alternatives, in part, because my aim is not to refute these views. My work provides supplementary resources that can be employed to augment alternatives such that they account for distinctive practices and goods realized through this valuable form of care. I have argued that perinatal hospice is valuable because it engages individuals, professional communities, and institutions in a common project of care that manifests virtues responsive to profound human need and vulnerability. Given the constructive aims of my work, consideration of alternatives can bring into relief some of the distinctive features of this *virtue-based* defense.

To begin, my defense is distinct from the *moral status* defense in two ways. First, it does not presuppose contested philosophical and theological doctrines concerning the moral status of the unborn child. A *virtue-based* defense can be developed and deployed by individuals who differ in their views on these vexed philosophical and theological issues. For those who reject the view that the unborn child is an individual with moral status, a *virtue-based* defense provides resources to account for the quality care provided for families who have chosen to continue the pregnancy. On this view, the scope of virtues such as hospitality extends to the family of the unborn child; it extends to the child only insofar as proper sensitivity to the family involves attending to ways the family thinks of their child as a beloved member of the family. For those who endorse the view that the unborn child has moral status, however, these virtues take the unborn child into their ambit of concern because of the child's moral status. Second, the *virtue-based* defense differs from the *moral status* defense in that it refuses to reduce the goods of this practice to the ways they uphold the child's moral worth. Perinatal hospice manifests a wide range of goods, many of which cannot be reduced to the ways that acknowledge or respect the value of the child.

It is also distinct from the *reproductive autonomy* defense in two ways. First, it does not reduce the value of perinatal hospice to the reproductive choices of families affected by an adverse *in utero* diagnosis. There are important goods manifested in this practice that are independent of the value of choice. This is especially the case if the unborn child has inherent moral status—a possibility that cannot be ruled out without substantive argument. As I noted in Chapter 1, the *reproductive autonomy* defense is committed to the view that the unborn child lacks inherent value. A *virtue-based* defense does not rule out this possibility *a priori*. Second, the *virtue-based* defense characterizes the value of perinatal hospice in terms of goods internal to the practice. Its value consists in the fact that it engages healthcare providers and institutions in a good common project that effectively addresses a family's needs for welcome, meaning, accompaniment, and consolation. The value of perinatal hospice is not reducible to the fact that it expands the range of choice options; its value is not dependent solely upon the respect it shows for the family's choice.

There is an additional difference worth noting in this context. Unlike the *moral status* and *reproductive autonomy* defenses, the *virtue-based* defense provides an account of the value of perinatal hospice that is separable from its status as an alternative to abortion. One can defend perinatal hospice as an ethical option in contexts where pregnancy termination is common, but its value does not consist solely in the fact that it offers an alternative to abortion. Defending perinatal hospice on its own terms involves attending to the goods realized in the practice, the structures and processes that manifest these goods, and the ways fitting care can provide meaning and fulfillment even in the midst of difficulty. An account of perinatal hospice that reduces its value to its status as an alternative to abortion fails to provide a clear portrait of this range of values. Most of my work in this book has been devoted to pointing to these values, goods, and exemplary care that manifests virtues.

This may address the differences between the *virtue-based* defense and the *moral status* and *reproductive* autonomy defenses respectively. But the differences between the *virtue-based* and the *supportive care* defense are worth extended attention because of some similarities in outlook and concern. The range of practices I have identified as expressive of virtue overlap with a number of practices proponents of the *supportive care* account identify as quality medical care. Furthermore, both views construe practices and social structures that inhibit the consideration of comfort-maximizing options as deficient. For these reasons, one may wonder whether the differences between the *virtue-based* defense and the *supportive care* defense are such that they provide reason to prefer one defense over the other.

I maintain that there are three primary differences between these accounts. First, they are grounded in distinct normative frameworks. The notion of fitting medical care implicit within the *supportive care* view is relatively thin compared to the robust virtue-theoretic framework I have articulated. According to the *supportive* care view, fitting medical care takes the best interest of the patient as its central focus. Physicians aim to provide care that is beneficial and displays mercy in providing for a patient's quality of life. They seek to ensure that interventions do not harm the patient. The *virtue-based* defense agrees that these are important ends, but it grounds them in a substantive framework concerning human fulfillment. According to this view, there are excellences crucial to human flourishing that take human need and vulnerability as a focal object of concern. The practices expressive of virtue and the professions and institutions that scaffold such care are those that properly attend to these needs. Even if these respective defenses identify some of the same basic practices and structures as morally commendable, the conceptual foundations supporting these judgments are distinct.

One may wonder whether a thin conceptual foundation better serves the defense of perinatal hospice. Given that accounts of human fulfillment often presuppose particular accounts of the nature of a good human life, a substantive *virtue-based* defense may require endorsing a robust metaphysical framework that limits its appeal. Appeals to quality care do not require this kind of commitment. Thus, a thin framework may be preferable because it requires one to endorse fewer contested views. But the *supportive care* view may require endorsing substantive commitments.

Notions such as the best interests of the patient, beneficent and merciful care, and quality of life may depend upon substantive metaphysical views. Thus, these appeals require further development and analysis. The advantage, then, of the *virtue-based* defense is that it makes explicit its metaphysical commitments at the outset while those implicit in the *supportive care* defense are left unanalyzed.

Second, the moral value of choice serves a distinct justificatory role in the respective accounts of the value of perinatal hospice. According to the *supportive care* defense, an attitude of deference is foundational to the support clinicians extend in the consideration of the continuance or termination of pregnancy. Additionally, the provision of perinatal hospice is valuable in part because it aligns medically appropriate care with family choices. Thus, both prior to the choice to continue the pregnancy and consequent upon this decision, choice serves a crucial justificatory function in its account of the value of perinatal hospice. Choice does not serve the same function in the *virtue-based* defense. On this view, perinatal hospice is valuable because it manifests virtue in its attention and care for the profound human needs of the child and the family. A family's choice to continue the pregnancy ensures that the family will experience distinct needs—needs that would not emerge if they chose to terminate the pregnancy. The value of perinatal hospice consists, in part, in the way it tends to these unique needs.

The fact the choice serves a different function in these respective analyses is not, by itself, a reason to prefer one over the other defense. But the fact that the goods manifested in the practice of perinatal hospice cannot be reduced to the value of choice suggests that an account of these goods needs to draw upon a framework where choice is not the only or the primary value served by the practice. The *supportive care* defense takes choice to be the fundamental value in the initial decision to continue or to terminate the pregnancy. The other values relevant in the context of care are consequent upon this initial choice. The *supportive care* view does not reduce these other values to the value of choice, but it makes their consideration secondary to whether the family makes a decision to continue the pregnancy.

Third, the *virtue-based* defense differs from the *supportive care* defense in its approach to the question of the moral status of the unborn child. According to the *supportive care* defense, the choice to continue the pregnancy establishes a ground for treating the unborn child as a patient. As a patient, the unborn child has interests that must be weighed in planning for its care. Prior to the decision to continue the pregnancy, however, clinicians must remain uncommitted concerning the question of the unborn child's moral status. Although this is a defensible position, it is not clear whether this account is compatible with the view that the unborn child has inherent moral worth. The fact that the unborn child's status as a patient depends completely upon the family's choice seems to imply that its moral status is derivative. But, for all one knows, moral status is inherent. It is not clear how the *supportive care* defense can countenance this possibility. In contrast, there are ways one can develop a *virtue-based* defense that are fully compatible with the possibility that the unborn child has inherent moral worth.

Extended reflection upon one of the virtues I have profiled in this work may suggest that we ought to consider this possibility with greater moral seriousness.[5] Part of the moral stance characteristic of the virtue of hospitality is its refusal to draw artificial boundaries between those outside and those within the moral community. Hospitable individuals and communities do not typically engage in the project of demarcating humans into groups of those who are deserving or undeserving of our care. Reflection upon the virtue of hospitality may thus encourage an expansive vision of who counts as a subject of moral concern—a vision that includes the unborn child as an individual with inherent worth and deserving of a hospitable welcome.[6] Although philosophical debates concerning moral status seem intractable, a defense of perinatal hospice should not foreclose *a priori* on the possibility the unborn child has inherent moral worth. Arguably, defenses of perinatal hospice that rule out such a possibility *a priori* fail to approach questions about the moral status of the unborn child with sufficient moral gravity.

One advantage of the substantive *virtue-based* framework I have developed in this work is that it enables one to countenance the possibility that the unborn child has intrinsic moral worth. But this framework may not be appealing to clinicians who wish to remain neutral on this vexed question. One may wish to develop a *virtue-based* framework that does not require specific consideration of contested philosophical issues. A thin *virtue-based* framework that restricts the scope of hospitality may have broader appeal. Such an account may defend perinatal hospice as an expression of hospitality to the family affected by an adverse *in utero* diagnosis while remaining neutral on the contested question of the moral status of the unborn child. But the broad appeal of such an account requires further defense because of the ways it narrows the expansive scope of hospitality's characteristic welcoming stance.

Contrasting a *virtue-based* defense of perinatal hospice with these alternatives highlights some of the distinctive features of my account. But I have not yet pointed to what I take to be its chief value as an account of the value of perinatal hospice: a *virtue-based* defense provides a substantive rationale for the claim that professional communities and medical institutions who desire to provide exemplary care ought to engage in a broad-based reform of deficient practices and social structures. Appeals to the moral status of the unborn child alone cannot ground the types of reforms I have identified in the conclusion of each chapter. Although they may ground reforms aimed at developing a more hospitable institutional culture, they will not be able to justify those reforms expressive of a culture of allocentric hope, solidarity, and compassion for the griefs of affective families. Likewise, appeals to reproductive autonomy are insufficient to justify the types of reforms I argued would create a culture of exemplary care. The fact that families choose to continue a pregnancy is not a sufficient basis for seeking to change institutional protocols in genetic counseling, in ensuring that families can exercise hope in difficult circumstances, in accompanying families through the difficulties of traversing multiple institutional spaces, and in addressing their needs for consolation. The *supportive care* view may provide some basis for these kinds of reform, but its initial deference to family choices and commitments may not provide a sufficient basis for the kinds of reform to genetic counseling and ensuring families feel welcomed into a space of care.

On the *virtue-based* defense I have developed, professional communities and medical institutions ought to engage in these reforms as a response to the summons of virtue to promote and provide exemplary care. These reforms are crucial because current practices and social structures fail to manifest virtue in the ways they address important human needs. Insofar as professional communities and their social structures fail to address human needs, they further undermine the chances that those with profound vulnerabilities can flourish. Thus, professional communities and institutions that fail to engage in this kind of reform fail to respond appropriately to tasks characteristic of virtue—that is, to the summons of virtue to excellence in caring for the needs of affected families. Social and structural deficiencies of the sort outlined in this work require social and structural remedies expressive of virtue. Professional communities ought to take up the tasks of promoting and providing this form of care. But are these tasks really possible in contemporary care settings? Do barriers to reform counsel against this pursuit? It is to these questions that I turn next.

III. Addressing Barriers to Reform

Throughout this work, I described a number of reforms that could help to address common needs following an adverse *in utero* diagnosis. Some of these reforms do not require significant cost or substantive institutional change, but others may involve serious efforts to make fundamental changes across various institutional levels within contemporary care settings. Reforms crucial to ensuring that perinatal hospice programs are widely available and accessible may require addressing both social structures external to medical institutions and widely shared commitments and beliefs that influence attitudes concerning the aims and value of medical practice.

Unfortunately, these tasks may be complicated by a wide range of obstacles. The primary aim of this section is to identify some of these barriers. Part of the commitment to engaging in a good common project of care involves addressing these factors.[7] Here, I focus on barriers associated with (i) lack of awareness, (ii) insufficient funding, (iii) politicization, and (iv) attitudinal commitments concerning the best ways to alleviate the burdens associated with suffering and disability.

First, consider those obstacles to care rooted in a lack of awareness of the needs of families and healthcare providers. The current infant mortality rate in the United States is approximately six deaths per 1,000 live births. Approximately 20% of infant deaths are attributable to congenital malformations and birth defects.[8] Many of these cases could benefit from palliative and hospice measures.[9] But perinatal hospice is a novel modality of care. It is not clear that healthcare providers and medical institutions are generally aware of the kinds of care they can make available. Furthermore, it is not clear that those working within NICUs have sufficient training in palliative and hospice care.

Professional communities and institutions are already seeking to address these obstacles through expanded efforts in education and training, but these attempts to address a lack of awareness are complicated by an institutional ethos ordered toward aggressive curative measures. In an extraordinarily technical and aggressive culture of care within the NICU, there is often a lack of training and experience in the provision of effective hospice care. As Wool (2013) notes,

> Clinicians in perinatal service lines do not, as a matter of routine, receive formal training in fetal [end-of-life] issues. As a result, there is wide variation in skills, knowledge, and beliefs as providers interface with parents who receive a life-limiting fetal diagnosis.
>
> (56)

Kain and Wilkinson (2013) acknowledge,

> There is often difficulty in accepting a palliative model of care in contemporary health care. There is a focus upon curative treatment regimens, with a drive to offer aggressive interventions. This may be because the serious nature of disease is still evolving or perhaps to postpone the acceptance that death has become inevitable. Health care needs to consider when no potentially curative intervention exists, or their benefits have become exhausted. This can lead to a feeling of hopelessness that there is nothing left to offer the newborn.
>
> (462)

Interestingly, the profitability of aggressive neonatal care may create further disincentives to the promotion and provision of perinatal hospice. As Meadow and Lantos (2009) observe:

> Neonatal intensive care is one of the most cost-effective tertiary care interventions in all of medicine. It is far more cost-effective than adult

intensive care, coronary bypass surgery, solid organ transplantation, renal dialysis, or many other well-accepted interventions. In standard economic approaches, treatments are considered cost-effective if they provide a quality-adjusted life- year (QALY) for less than $50,000. In neonatology, each QALY costs less than $10,000 even for infants at the lowest birth weights. Put another way, in the NICU, at least 90 cents of every dollar spent is devoted to an infant who will survive to go home.

(595)

When one combines these successes with the reality that most private and public health insurance schemes cover neonatal intensive care, the NICU can provide a substantive economic benefit to medical institutions.[10] In fact, the profitability of the NICU has led to the proliferation of these units across the nation. The increasing availability of NICU technology combined with the increasing numbers of physicians and advanced practice nurses with specializations in these areas may entrench tendencies toward overtreatment.[11] In short, economic variables can incentivize a culture of aggressive care, undercutting support for the promotion and provision of perinatal hospice.

Furthermore, healthcare providers may struggle because of sociocultural attitudes concerning the aims of medicine in relation to death and suffering. Recommending hospice care when lives of vulnerable children hang in the balance seems like a failure, a capitulation to an eventuality that medicine promised one could forestall or prevent. Kain and Wilkinson (2013) write,

> At a societal level, death and dying in infancy is driven by high emotional content because the death of a newborn is considered a life that has ended too soon: illness and death are unexpected for a newborn and are devastating and life-altering events for the family. Society in general does not know how to respond to the death of a newborn, and therefore have few established social norms to help a family cope with such loss. Society more readily accepts deaths of adults and even of children. Complicating these ethical concerns is the notion that the death of a newborn in this highly curative environment is a failure of medical science.
>
> (462)

Acceptance of the limits of medical care requires a kind of acquiescence that is foreign to the typical ethos and dramatic success of the NICU unit. In these contexts, healthcare providers may struggle to care for families because they perceive themselves as failing to deliver on the promise of medical care.

It may take some time to address these attitudes concerning the aims of medical care, but the best way to achieve reforms in this domain is to ensure that healthcare providers benefit from an education and enculturation within clinical practice that includes exposure to the delivery of palliative and hospice care. In addition to this, specific training in engaging with families concerning difficult questions of advanced care planning can facilitate greater comfort in discussing end-of-life care.[12] Reforms in education and training of this sort will create opportunities for healthcare providers to evaluate their own attitudes concerning the ultimate aims of medicine. It will help them to cultivate a better appreciation for the limitations of their practice. Hopefully, it will increase their sensitivity to and willingness to own these limitations in the pursuit of palliative aims when these are appropriate.

Second, consider those obstacles to care rooted in insufficient funding for perinatal hospice. At times, these barriers are related to failures in communication channels. The financial administrators within medical institutions may be unaware of the need for additional funds for the specific provision of palliative and hospice care.[13] This is compounded by uncertainties concerning costs of care and insurance coverage. At present, most private insurance covers palliative and hospice care for children; government insurance programs typically cover these costs as well.[14] But this may not be common knowledge. Failures to communicate this information to families or delays in determining coverage may inhibit full consideration of palliative options.

There are other barriers related to uncovered costs: coverage of the insured does not account for costs associated with the uninsured or the underinsured; it does not account for potential costs associated with advanced care-planning especially if these are not billable; and it does not address the costs associated with the commitment required of those who seek to be present to these families. A recent profile of Dr. Conrad Williams, program director of pediatric palliative care at Medical University of South Carolina (MUSC), offers a clear portrait of this particular funding challenge:

> As the pediatric palliative care team's medical director, [Williams] must figure out how to float a program that doesn't generate a profit for his employer. MUSC, and thousands of other hospitals in the United States, tie physician salaries to productivity—how many patients they treat and how many surgeries they perform. But Williams does little of that. At work, he mainly talks to people. No medical billing codes exist for sending a condolence card or attending a funeral. And while he's convinced that pediatric palliative care is meaningful, even essential, for children and their families, he also understands, from the hospital's perspective, that it's not lucrative. He gives MUSC credit for spending money it knows it won't get back. "Two days ago, I was with a family, pretty much all day, at the end of life," he said recently. "In a month, I could come back and tell you what I actually was able to bill from that—from a money

standpoint—and what we actually collected, based on spending four or five hours with that family and documenting that encounter. It's probably going to be a few hundred bucks." That won't come close to covering his salary and benefits. "In the eyes of the numbers people in the hospital system," he admitted, "that doesn't make a lot of financial sense."[15]

Noting these difficulties, Williams acknowledges that he must engage in external fundraising to ensure adequate provision of pediatric palliative care. If funding for these programs depends upon the efforts of caregivers who seek external sources of financing, their sustainability may be difficult to secure. Furthermore, if financial support for these programs issues primarily from sources external to the institution, administrators may display an unwillingness to commit to funding these programs as a part of the institution's annual budgetary commitments.

Addressing these financial obstacles will require sustained efforts of both private and public institutions. A central part of this collective endeavor may involve systematic efforts to remove uncertainties in the coverage of the costs for both advanced care planning and the provision of palliative and hospice care. Some may seek to ensure that private insurance specifically covers perinatal hospice as a form of care. Others may advance legislation to encourage state and federal insurance programs to cover these costs. In addition to this, communities may need to promote charitable donations to established programs of care so that they can address unmet needs.[16]

These activities may not be sufficient in contexts where one must factor the potential costs of perinatal hospice against the expenses associated with the termination of pregnancy. As Lantos and Meadow (2011) observe, "From a purely economic perspective, termination of pregnancy is very cost-effective. Babies who are not born alive do not require expensive neonatal care" (196). Although the potential costs of perinatal hospice are substantially less than aggressive neonatal intensive care, they are potentially much higher than the cost of abortion. Given the legal status of abortion and the potentially high costs of care for perinatal hospice, medical institutions may be disinclined to promote or provide perinatal hospice.

Questions about the costs of care and proper distribution of resources are appropriate, but endorsing this moral calculus requires adopting the perspective that the financial costs of caring for child with a significantly life-limiting condition justify ending his life prior to birth. This is problematic, in part, because it requires reducing the value of the unborn child's life to an economic variable. Considerations of virtuous care must be distinguished from this kind of unqualified economic reasoning. Furthermore, given the financial pressures facing medical institutions, healthcare providers and professional communities must be attentive to the ways both institutional policies and protocols and their own decisions are influenced by these kinds of economic considerations. Termination of pregnancy may be less expensive than perinatal hospice, but this is not a sufficient reason to pressure families to choose abortion. At a minimum, this kind of calculation fails to consider the potential that the unborn child's value cannot be reduced to economic values. Financial administrators, in particular, must ensure that their decisions concerning care are not based solely upon the comparative economic costs of perinatal hospice and abortion.[17]

Third, consider the barriers to the promotion and provision of perinatal hospice grounded in the politically divisive issue of abortion. Earlier, I noted how legal restrictions on abortion choice can alter encounters between healthcare providers and affected families. Given that many jurisdictions place restrictions on abortive procedures at advanced stages of pregnancy, healthcare providers and families often experience an increased sense of urgency in making decisions following an adverse diagnosis. These legal structures may be a contributing factor to the overt and subtle pressures to terminate the pregnancy.

But this is not the only barrier to a full consideration of perinatal hospice; there are additional obstacles emerging from the politicization of perinatal hospice in recent legislative efforts. Recall that initial defenses of perinatal hospice focused primarily on its function as an alternative to abortion. As a result, public advocacy of perinatal hospice in the United States has been aimed at ensuring that affected families have access to information concerning this form of care. Some have sought to introduce legislation predicated on the view that awareness of perinatal hospice is essential for the family to make an informed decision following diagnosis. At present, there are several states (including Arizona, Indiana, Kansas, Minnesota, Mississippi, and Oklahoma) that have passed legislation of this sort. A number of other state legislatures have considered perinatal hospice legislation. Opponents of these legislative efforts argue that these efforts are thinly veiled attempts to curtail abortion rights. They add that these measures often compound the emotional burdens families experience by stigmatizing the private decision to terminate the pregnancy.[18]

Thus, one potential barrier to the promotion and provision of perinatal hospice is the perception that public advocacy of these programs of care is best construed as a political weapon in the culture wars concerning abortion. What gets lost in the process is an awareness and appreciation of the ways these programs manifest virtue in addressing the needs of families. The politicization of perinatal hospice threatens to undermine alliances between individuals across the political spectrum crucial to the promotion and provision of these virtuous forms of care.

Addressing these political barriers may require proponents of perinatal hospice to adopt a different political strategy. By promoting perinatal hospice as an alternative to abortion, or as crucial to making informed decisions following an adverse diagnosis, or as a vital support to women in contexts where there are societal pressures to terminate the pregnancy, advocates appear to be promoting perinatal hospice as a plank within an overarching political agenda. Politicizing the promotion of perinatal hospice in this way will not convince those who are wary of this broad political agenda. Thus, political efforts to expand awareness of and access to perinatal hospice should move beyond an exclusive focus on legislation tethered to informed consent provisions in abortion statutes. As I note elsewhere, a compelling positive case for broad public support of perinatal hospice should involve

> identifying the goods internal to these practices and embedding them within a broad account of the ways in which these practices are constitutive of a flourishing community. What these forms of care make available are avenues to address real human needs; a community that offers perinatal hospice is a community that seeks to foster a virtuous response in the midst of harrowing circumstances.
>
> (Cobb 2016, 36)

Political efforts ought to focus on increasing awareness of and funding for these caregiving practices and the ways they address needs. Proponents of perinatal hospice can lobby to ensure that both private and public health insurance covers the costs of care. If individuals continue to pursue legislative efforts to promote perinatal hospice, these attempts ought to be conjoined to significant attempts to secure public and private investments such that these programs are widely available and adequately supported. Political advocacy for perinatal hospice must focus on goods internal to the practice and not merely on the practices to which it provides an alternative.

Fourth, and finally, consider the barriers that are rooted in societal attitudes and commitments concerning burdens associated with suffering and disability. There are many who assume that termination of an affected pregnancy is the best way to address the suffering of the family. In a recent study, Wool (2013) found that

> physicians perceived termination to be a more healing alternative than [perinatal palliative care], differing significantly with their nurse colleagues. Perhaps this stems from a notion that termination of the pregnancy provides parents with more immediate closure, thus allowing them to move into a healing process sooner. Physicians also differed with nurses in believing continuation of a pregnancy may place an undue emotional burden on families.
>
> (55)

To the extent that these physicians' attitudes are mirrored within the broader culture and the family's personal community, the family may think of abortion as a remedy to potential suffering. Given that "the availability of termination obligates parents to accept or refuse it as an option" (Wool and Dudek 2013, 534), they may choose to terminate the pregnancy in order to prevent their suffering.

Similarly, some assume that the burdens of living with a profound disability are so great that it would be better to prevent the child from being born. Meadow and Lantos (2009) note that physicians often struggle with distress over the fact that advances in neonatal intensive care have caused families to bear the burden of care for a child with significant morbidities. They comment that the most common factor contributing to this distress is "guilt over the long-term implications for families when a neurologically devastated infant survives" (596). They note that "the worst outcome of neonatology is not death in the NICU but the long-term survival of a neurologically devastated infant" (2009, 596). Physicians struggle to reconcile the success of neonatal intensive care with the fact that these practices are partly responsible for causing children and their families to experience added burdens. In light of these attitudes, the availability of a means by which families can alleviate these burdens prior to birth may contribute to a physician's felt need to counsel against continuing the pregnancy. If the lives of individuals with significantly life-limiting conditions are suboptimal and families can be kept from experiencing these burdens, this may be a sufficient rationale for terminating the pregnancy.[19]

These kinds of barriers are perhaps the most difficult to address; it is difficult to budge broadly shared attitudes and commitments concerning the perceived burdens of suffering and disability. But there are important reasons to challenge some of the assumptions implicit in the views articulated here. It is not clear, for instance, that healthcare providers are sufficiently sensitive to the evidence that their judgments concerning the value of disabled lives do not always match the judgments of individuals with these disabilities or the judgments of their families.[20]

It is also not clear whether these attitudes and commitments reflect sufficient appreciation of the gravity of the family's suffering following the choice to terminate a pregnancy. There is a range of evidence suggesting that abortion may not alleviate or diminish the family's suffering. In a recent systematic analysis of evidence concerning the psychological sequelae of termination for reasons of fetal anomaly, Sullivan and Faoite (2017) note that this decision opens women up to a wide range of psychological effects including posttraumatic stress disorder, anxiety, and depression. Their review of ten recent studies revealed that although

> these studies differ in size, scope, and intent, it is clear that induced abortion following the prenatal diagnosis of a potentially deadly foetal anomaly can take a devastating toll on the mothers who receive the news and then must make the difficult decision of whether to terminate or continue with the pregnancy until birth.

(25–26)

These effects can be both severe and long-lasting. Sullivan and Faoite (2017) conclude that healthcare providers "advising patients to abort in an effort to avoid unnecessary or excess psychological turmoil may be proposing a counterproductive solution" (27).[21]

If this is correct, then healthcare providers who direct (or implicitly pressure) families to terminate the pregnancy because they see it as the compassionate choice, or the only choice that effectively alleviates suffering, or as the best option for addressing potential emotional burdens, fail to display proper seriousness in their care for a family who must make a complicated, life-altering choice. Care for the family must take seriously the potential suffering they may experience because of a choice to terminate the pregnancy. It must take into account the evidence that continuing the pregnancy may have beneficial effects for the family. As Coleman (2015) notes,

> Studies addressing the psychological experiences of women who chose not to terminate . . . are tending to indicate that these women experience less suffering than women who terminate their pregnancies. In fact there is evidence indicating that women who continue their pregnancies are inclined to derive some meaning from the experience, often reporting positive insights and emotions associated with the pregnancy and birth.
>
> (15)

One recent study, for instance, suggests that very few families who make the choice to continue a pregnancy experience regret concerning their decision. Wool, Limbo, and Denney-Koelsch (2018) report that, in a study of 402 individuals who continued the pregnancy following an adverse diagnosis, 97.5% indicated that they had no regrets about this decision (229–230). Of the ten individuals who expressed some regrets, only three offered qualitative responses concerning the nature of these regrets. None of them expressed regrets concerning the choice to continue the pregnancy; their regrets focused on decisions about care following birth or inadequate pain control for the child.

Both personal and professional communities may suggest to the family that terminating the pregnancy is the best they could do in the circumstances; it is the best of a bad lot of choices. For the family, considering this choice requires attending to the serious nature of its moral implications. The family must recognize that this choice will change them; it will require them to embrace a distinct kind of suffering. They will have to integrate both their grief in the loss of the child and the additional burden of knowing that they chose to bring about this loss.[22] There is potential for moral residue in reconciling the choice to their sense of self and moral identity. Given the concern for how they might be perceived by others, these individuals may experience this sorrow in private, outside the supportive care of a community of family and friends.

The promotion and provision of perinatal hospice can enable families to see that there are ways to address their concerns for the suffering of the child, or their inability to provide care sufficient to address the child's pain, or to bear their own suffering in circumstances of profound need. If the unborn child has a significantly life-limiting condition, it does not follow that he is actively suffering, or that his future suffering will be so devastating that it cannot be addressed. In fact, in many cases, the child does not suffer. At birth, he may have profound limitations and needs, but there are forms of care that can minimize pain and suffering. Given the advances in palliative medicine, many children who are born with life-limiting conditions will die peacefully in the loving care of their families.

The aim of this section was to identify and address some of the chief challenges to the creation and promotion of perinatal programs. There are barriers rooted in a lack of awareness, insufficient funding, politicization, and entrenched attitudes concerning the proper ways to address the burdens associated with suffering and disability. Although I treated these barriers separately, they interact and reinforce each other in varied ways within the contemporary care setting. They may inhibit the cultivation of a hospitable, hopeful, solidary, and compassionate ethos of medical care. But if the *virtue-based* defense I have developed is well-grounded, communities who seek to address these barriers for the sake of affected families engage in an exemplary form of virtuous care. Failure to engage in this project constitutes a failure to exhibit a proper sensitivity to and vigilant care for the concerns of virtue. It is a failure to respond to the summons of virtue to provide exemplary care.

IV. Conclusion—The Personal Is the Philosophical Is the Political

Questions about the ethics of end-of-life care are complicated. They are even more difficult when they concern human life in its earliest stages. Developments in and the increasing use of prenatal screening, have created novel moral questions for families facing the difficult prospects of caring for a child with a significantly life-limiting condition. I have argued that perinatal hospice is a common project of care that can address the real needs of families who choose to continue an affected pregnancy. Although this chapter shows that the reforms crucial to realizing these goods may be difficult in the short term, the narratives throughout this work show that there are individuals, professional communities, and institutions already engaged in common projects of this sort. Even in those contexts where there are no structured programs, there are ways to ensure that families benefit from this exemplary approach to care. Given the commitments I enumerated in Chapter 1, it is fitting to draw this work to a close by reflecting on the ways my family benefitted from the care of a professional community in a setting where there were no structured perinatal hospice programs. This kind of narrative offers some hope that professional communities can be moved to respond to need even in contexts where formal structures for the promotion and provision of this care do not yet exist.

Earlier I noted that families who receive an adverse *in utero* diagnosis often report feeling unwelcomed by the physicians and institutions from whom they hope to receive care. This was our own experience when dealing with the fetal and maternal health specialists who diagnosed Samuel. Early in the pregnancy, we knew that Sam was facing significant challenges. An ultrasound around thirteen weeks into the pregnancy indicated that he had an omphalocele. Additional testing at seventeen and twenty weeks confirmed that Sam had trisomy 18 along with a range of associated anomalies. The physician informed us that the most likely outcome was *in utero* demise; if he made it to birth, his life was likely to be very short and significantly difficult. He was not a candidate for active interventions after birth. She noted that we could interrupt the pregnancy; if we chose to continue the pregnancy, she claimed that there was nothing they would be able to do for us. At that point, she left us alone, stating that she would return in a few minutes to receive our decision. In the clinical space of an examination room detached from friends and family, we were left alone to determine what we would like to do.

There are a number of ways we could interpret this encounter. Perhaps her words were a simple acknowledgement that this particular institution did not offer any forms of care for children like Sam. Perhaps there was a desire to ensure that we understood that trisomy 18 was an incurable condition. She may have thought that we were under the mistaken impression that it could be healed. Perhaps she hoped that communicating in this way would help us to retrain our attention on my wife to ensure that she had adequate care.

I do not wish to impute vice to the particular physician who had the awful task of communicating a devastating diagnosis to our family. This was a brief consultation—probably one of several she had on this day and, more likely than not, an interaction governed by protocols for engagement with families like ours. The fact that we only had a few minutes to make this decision may have been standard procedure within this institutional setting. Furthermore, institutional protocols were likely structured by factors beyond her control. Given the legal constraints in our jurisdiction, it was important to communicate the need for a timely decision. Taken together, all of these constraints may have led her to adopt the kind of clinical detachment we perceived in our interactions with her.

Contrast this with the way in which my wife's obstetrician received us. At our first visit one week after diagnosis, she sat with us and asked, "What can I do to help you honor your time with Samuel?" She worked with us to craft a plan for care in the event that he made it to birth—a plan she eventually communicated directly to the nursing staff at the NICU and to the neonatologist who cared for Sam. She scheduled standing weekly appointments so we could hear his heartbeat or see his frame on an ultrasound. She allowed us to enter the back door so we would not have to sit with other families who were unaware of what we were experiencing. We were able to include our four-year-old son on one of these visits. He was able to see his brother on the ultrasound. What we experienced from her, her partners, her nursing staff, and eventually the entire labor and delivery and NICU team was the experience of institutional care. We were not left outside on the threshold; we were invited in. They were individually and collectively attuned to our need for welcome; through their care, they manifested the virtue of hospitality.

Our own experience also shows the role of personal and professional communities in the maintenance of our hopes. The fact that my wife's obstetrician helped us honor our time with Sam provided a foundation for our ongoing hope. We knew he would not live long after birth; there were too many complications. But the consistent weekly appointments enabled us to acknowledge his ongoing presence with us. As the weeks stretched on, we were able to cling to our hopes to meet him, to be able to hold him, and to be able to introduce him to family and friends. The maternal-fetal specialists who communicated Sam's grim prognosis to us failed to perceive or imagine how the investment in these hopes could endow the experience with great meaning. At the time of decision, we did not fully appreciate this fact either. It was the sustained provision of care that enabled us to see the value in the care we received.

Our family, friends, and colleagues rallied to underscore the significance of our calling to care for Samuel. Even if none of our residual hopes were realized, their presence assured us that there was great meaning in persevering in this pursuit. We could hope to fulfill this calling even if none of the concrete outcomes for which we hoped came to fruition. The provision of care made possible by the professional community of healthcare providers made it possible for our personal community to join in the project of sustaining us in hope.

I have already noted some of the key ways in which healthcare providers were present to us, accompanying us in our pursuit of these limited hopes. There were no official perinatal hospice programs in Alabama at the time. So, we worked to create a plan of care, borrowing ideas we discovered through research and conversation with friends. We communicated our desires to our obstetrician. Part of me wondered whether we were doing all that we could, whether we were adequately attending to our four-year-old son's needs, whether the NICU would know what we needed if my wife's obstetrician was not available. I remember finding this process emotionally taxing given our already present grief. An official perinatal hospice program with a central coordinator and structured system would have offered a kind of accompaniment that could have enhanced our experience during the wait. It would have relieved some anxiety and offered us a deeper sense that we were doing well to provide for our sons. But, in spite of these difficulties, we did not feel abandoned; we were supported well throughout the experience.

My family was fortunate to have a good community of friends and family who were present to us as well. Many of our deepest and most important relationships were forged and strengthened in these circumstances. Our community did not leave us alone; they came near and remained with us. This kind of good fortune is rare; there are many who feel abandoned both by healthcare providers and institutions and by their personal communities.

When the time came for Sam's delivery, our experience at the hospital was beautiful and profoundly meaningful. From my wife's obstetrician to the neonatologist to the nurses and the nurse practitioner who were working in the NICU, we had a joyful and significant five hours with our son. The care we received both immediately after his birth and throughout his short life was both supportive and kind. The nurses enabled us to experience his life as something beautiful, sacred, and, surprisingly, normal. I held my son for almost the entirety of the five hours he was with us. We were able to introduce him to friends. Our pastor was present to baptize him. In his final moments, everyone huddled around him and prayed together through tears. After his death, the nurses carefully cleaned him and brought his body to us in my wife's recovery room. We were able to stay with him and to say our final goodbyes. All of these final acts have been crucial to our ongoing healing as we grieve.

We knew we could not hope for a long life. But we hoped to pour as much love as possible into Sam's life while he lived. The physicians and nurses along with our personal community made it possible for us to fulfill these hopes and more. In their commitment to a common project of care, they helped us to see the meaning and significance of our choice to welcome Samuel. Shortly after my son's death, I wrote these words to capture the ways this professional community facilitated the experience of deep meaning in the midst of grief:

> Four hours and fifty-eight minutes—the official length of his life. For most of that time, I held my son, my sweet Samuel. His weak and frail body, his sweet cry, his dark eyes—I studied him. And he watched me. I could do nothing but hold him, listen to him, let him hear my voice, let his eyes catch mine. In these hours, I felt the weight of love in his three pound, twelve ounce frame. I experienced the depth of love as I covered him with smiles and tears. I felt the grace of friendship as I welcomed him into a loving community. I saw myself in my son. I saw my own helplessness reflected in his eyes; I recognized my own vulnerability in his brokenness. Life unites us; so does dying. And he died looking directly into my eyes. I kissed his

forehead and he was gone. A blink, a breath, a whisper—the entirety of a life. And these moments have forever altered my understanding of significance.

(Cobb 2014, 38–9)

By promoting and providing these forms of care, professional communities can respond to needs that are at the heart of virtuous concern. By welcoming families and their unborn children, they express a concern at the heart of the virtue of hospitality. By helping to sustain the family's sense of meaning and possibility, they express a concern at the heart of the virtue of hope. By accompanying families as they wait, they express a concern at the heart of the virtue of solidarity. By consoling the family in their varied griefs, they express a concern at the heart of the virtue of compassion.

Perinatal hospice is a common project of care expressive of virtue, vital to addressing profound human needs. This is its central and abiding value. Thus, individual healthcare providers, professional communities, medical institutions, and our local communities ought to promote and provide this kind of exemplary care.

Notes

1 MacIntyre (1999) call these traits virtues of acknowledged dependence.
2 I'm grateful to my friend Craig Boyd for helping me to appreciate the ecstatic quality of these virtues.
3 For discussion of common projects, see Adams (2006).
4 In Chapter 2, I briefly noted a fourth approach—a virtue-based approach grounded in an empirical survey of physician and family perspectives on quality care. Although there is continuity between these accounts, I enumerated a number of differences earlier in this work. For this reason, I do not detail the differences here.
5 In her work on virtue theory and abortion, Rosalind Hursthouse (1991) argues that abstract philosophical theorizing concerning moral status is irrelevant to a morally serious appraisal of abortion. But sympathetic critics of Hursthouse's account have raised objections concerning her treatment of the issue of moral status. Kornegay (2011) contends that Hursthouse's discussion of cases where abortion is permissible presupposes a view according to which "the status of the fetus is lower than that of a typical adult or an infant" (55) and "the fetus's status grows in significance as it develops" (55). Hacker-Wright (2007) claims, "Hursthouse is not setting aside the issue of moral status in her treatment of the issue of abortion, but implicitly pursuing a very different way of thinking about the matter" (450). For additional criticism, see Lu (2011).
6 It is worth noting that families who choose to terminate an affected pregnancy do not find themselves in an inhospitable environment for these choices. This kind of welcome is an already common and established practice within medical institutions, professional communities, and the broader culture.
7 The literature on perinatal palliative and hospice care suggests that there are a wide range of barriers. I can highlight only a few in this context. For further

discussion, see Carter (2018); Denney-Koelsch et al. (2016); Kain (2006); Kain and Wilkinson (2013); Korzeniewska-Eksterowicz et al. (2013); Limbo et al. 2017; Williams-Reade et al. (2015); Wool (2013, 2015); Wool and Dudek (2013); Wool et al. (2016); and Wool, Limbo, and Denney-Koelsch (2018).

8 For details, see www.cdc.gov/reproductivehealth/MaternalInfantHealth/InfantMortality.htm (accessed 11/21/2018).

9 For helpful discussion of these issues in the context of pediatric palliative care, see Field and Behrman (2003)

10 Lantos and Meadow (2006) note that,

> [a]fter the Baby Doe controversy, in which the federal government tried to mandate treatment of almost all newborns, it became difficult to imagine a public policy in the United States that would allow care to be systematically limited. Instead, the opposite happened. Public policies were enacted that generously reimbursed NICUs. This led to a different sort of economic calculus for NICUs, one that focuses not on overall societal expenditures and societal benefits but that instead looks at the fiscal realities of individual hospitals and the doctors who work there. In our decentralized health care system, these economic forces are much more powerful drivers of actual behavior than the theoretical calculations of societal costs and benefits.
> (129)

For further discussion, see Lantos and Meadow (2006, 2011); Meadow and Lantos (2009); Meadow et al. (2012a, 2012b); and Muraskas and Parsi (2008).

11 For further discussion, see Camosy (2010).

12 See Wool (2013) for further discussion.

13 In a recent ethnography, Williams-Reade et al. (2015) studied the distinct clinical, operational, and financial dimensions of care within an institution that was seeking to implement a perinatal palliative care program. They discovered a number of barriers including difficulties in communication within and across team members as well as inadequate lines of communication between clinicians and those in charge of the financial decisions tied to the delivery of care.

14 For further discussion, see Field and Behrman (2003) and Keim-Malpass, Hart, and Miller (2013). In the United Kingdom, the National Health Service (NHS) provides statutory funding for a portion of the costs of hospice: adult hospice care receives approximately 30% of its funding from the NHS; children's hospices receive, on average, approximately 15% of its funding from statutory provisions. The remainder of care is from private and charitable organizations. For details of this funding as well as an articulation of the difficulties of funding hospice in a distinct regulatory framework, see: www.hospiceuk.org/about-hospice-care/media-centre/press-releases/details/2015/07/13/fragile-outlook-on-statutory-funding-for-hospices-in-england (accessed November 21, 2018).

15 For an extended discussion, see www.postandcourier.com/health/how-a-charleston-pediatrician-helps-children-at-the-end-of/article_1dbf81ca-cbcc-11e7-9830-9b499335fdd7.html (accessed on March 14, 2018).

16 For a current list of programs, see www.perinatalhospice.org/list-of-programs. Guimarães et al. (2019) describes the development of a new program in Portugal.

17 Likewise, their decisions should not be a function of economic incentives. Aggressive treatments may help to drive the profitability of the institution, but this is not a sufficient reason to preempt a consideration of comfort-maximizing care.

18 Similar political dynamics are at play in other jurisdictions. Consider, for instance, the 2018 referendum vote on the Eighth Amendment in Ireland. Advocates for repeal noted a discrepancy in care for families who received an adverse *in utero* diagnosis. Given the legal protections for unborn human life established by the Eighth Amendment, families who chose to terminate the pregnancy had to travel out of country to receive medical care. Advocates for repeal argued that the repeal would benefit women who chose to terminate the pregnancy because they would no longer experience the burdens of seeking care elsewhere. For a representative discussion, see www.irishtimes.com/news/ireland/irish-news/abortion-debate-eighth-creates-inequalities-in-foetal-abnormalities-care-1.3502060 (accessed November 21, 2018). Opponents of the repeal argued that Ireland ought to expand funding for perinatal hospice programs rather than extending the legal permissions for abortion. For a representative example, see www.thejournal.ie/love-both-hospice-3978097-Apr2018/ (accessed November 21, 2018). Advocates for repeal countered that their support for expanded legal options for abortion were not exclusive of expanded support for perinatal hospice.

19 For further discussion of disability and its import for the ethics of prenatal screening and abortion, see Asch and Wasserman (2005); Brock (2005); Kittay and Kittay (2000); Reinders (2000); Watt (2017).

20 For some discussion, see Janvier, Farlow, and Wilfond (2012); Janvier and Watkins (2013); McCaffrey (2016); and Saigal et al. (1999).

21 Some of the earlier discussion in this book may offer a plausible explanation for why families who choose to terminate an affected pregnancy may experience some of these adverse psychological outcomes. First, many of these families receive a diagnosis at an advanced stage of fetal gestation. This represents an interruption of a wanted pregnancy and a desired child. The losses attending this diagnosis by itself may induce grief. Second, families who choose to terminate may experience additional adverse effects because their choice diminishes opportunities for social validation of parental identity and for caregiving opportunities. Families who grieve the loss of the child they choose to abort may experience further complications or disenfranchisement in their grief because they lack these kinds of support.

22 For some discussion of the complicated nature of choice following prenatal diagnosis, see Benute et al. (2012); Bijma, van der Heide, and Wildschut (2008); Sandelowski and Barroso (2005); and Sandelowski and Jones (1996).

References

Adams, Robert. 2006. *A Theory of Virtue: Excellence in Being for the Good.* Oxford: Clarendon Press.

Asch, Adrienne and David Wasserman. 2005. "Where is the Sin in Synecdoche?" In *Quality of Life and Human Difference: Genetic Testing, Healthcare and Disability*, edited by David Wasserman, Robert Wachbroit, and Jerome Bickenbach, 172–216. Cambridge: Cambridge University Press.

Benute, Gláucia R.G., Roseli M.Y. Nomura, Adolfo W. Liao, Maria de Lourdes Brizot, Mara de Lucia, and M. Zugaib. 2012. "Feelings of Women Regarding End-of-life Decision Making after Ultrasound Diagnosis of a Lethal Fetal Malformation." *Midwifery* 28 (4): 472–5.

Bijma, Hilmar H., Agnes van der Heide, and Hajo IJ Wildschut. 2008. "Decision-making After Ultrasound Diagnosis of Fetal Abnormality." *Reproductive Health Matters* 16 (31): 82–9.

Brock, Dan M. 2005. "Preventing Genetically Transmitted Disabilities While Respecting Persons with Disabilities." In *Quality of Life and Human Difference: Genetic Testing, Healthcare and Disability*, edited by David Wasserman, Robert Wachbroit, and Jerome Bickenbach, 67–100. Cambridge: Cambridge University Press.

Camosy, Charles C. 2010. *Too Expensive To Treat? Finitude, Tragedy, and the Neonatal ICU*. Grand Rapids, MI: Wm. B. Eerdmans Publishing.

Carter, Brian S. 2018. "Pediatric Palliative Care in Infants and Neonates." *Children* 5 (2): 21–9.

Cobb, Aaron D. 2014. *Loving Samuel: Suffering, Dependence, and the Calling of Love*. Eugene: Cascade Books.

Cobb, Aaron D. 2016. "Acknowledged Dependence and the Virtues of Perinatal Hospice." *Journal of Medicine and Philosophy* 41 (1): 25–40.

Coleman, Priscilla K. 2015. "Diagnosis of Fetal Anomaly and the Increased Maternal Psychological Toll Associated with Pregnancy Termination." *Issues in Law & Medicine* 30 (1): 3–23.

Denney-Koelsch, Erin, Beth Perry Black, Denise Côté-Arsenault, Charlotte Wool, Sujeong Kim, and Karen Kavanaugh. 2016. "A Survey of Perinatal Palliative Care Programs in the United States: Structure, Processes, and Outcomes." *Journal of Palliative Medicine* 19 (10): 1080–6.

Field, Marilyn J. and Richard E. Behrman. 2003. *When Children Die: Improving Palliative and End-of-Life Care for Children and Their Families*. Washington, DC: National Academies Press.

Guimarães, Diana Paula Gomes, Maria Hercília Ferreira Guimarães Pereira Areias, Carla Maria de Almeida Ramalho, Maria Manuela Rodrigues. 2019. "Perinatal Palliative Care Following Prenatal Diagnosis of Severe Fetal Anomaly: A New Family-centered Approach in a Level III Portuguese Hospital." *Journal of Pediatric and Neonatal Individualized Medicine* 8 (1): online first.

Hacker-Wright, John. 2007. "Moral Status in Virtue Ethics." *Philosophy* 82 (3): 449–73.

Hursthouse, Rosalind. 1991. "Virtue Theory and Abortion." *Philosophy and Public Affairs* 20 (3): 223–46.

Janvier, Annie and Andrew Watkins. 2013. "Medical Interventions for Children with Trisomy 13 and Trisomy 18: What is the Value of a Short Disabled Life?" *Acta Paediatrica* 102 (12): 1112–17.

Janvier, Annie, Barbara Farlow, and Benjamin S. Wilfond. 2012. "The Experience of Families with Children with Trisomy 13 an 18 in Social Networks." *Pediatrics* 130 (2): 293–8.

Kain, Victoria J. and Dominic J. Wilkinson. 2013. "Neonatal Palliative Care in Action: Moving Beyond the Rhetoric and Influencing Policy." *Journal of Research in Nursing* 18 (5): 459–68.

Kain, Victoria. 2006. "Palliative Care Delivery in the NICU: What Barriers do Neonatal Nurses Face?" *Neonatal Network* 25 (6): 387–92.

Keim-Malpass, Jessica, Terra G. Hart, and Joy R. Miller. 2013. "Coverage of Palliative and Hospice Care for Pediatric Patients with a Life-limiting Illness: A Policy Brief." *Journal of Pediatric Health Care* 27 (6): 511–16.

Kittay, Eva Feder and Leo Kittay. 2000. "On the Expressivity and Ethics of Selective Abortion for disability: Conversations with My Son." In *Prenatal Testing and Disability Rights*, edited by Erik Parens and Adrienne Asch, 165–94. Washington, DC: Georgetown University Press.

Kornegay, R. Jo. 2011. "Hursthouse's Virtue Ethics and Abortion: Abortion Ethics without Metaphysics?" *Ethical Theory and Moral Practice* 14 (1): 51–71.

Korzeniewska-Eksterowicz, Aleksandra, Maria Respondek-Liberska, Łukasz Przysło, Wojciech Fendler, Wojciech Młynarski, and Ewa Gulczyńska. 2013. "Perinatal Palliative Care: Barriers and Attitudes of Neonatologists and Nurses in Poland." *The Scientific World Journal* 2013: 1–7.

Lantos, John D. and William L. Meadow. 2011. "Costs and End-of-life Care in the NICU: Lessons for the MICU?" *Journal of Law, Medicine & Ethics* 39 (2): 194–200.

Lantos, John D. and William L. Meadow. 2006. *Neonatal Bioethics: The Moral Challenges of Medical Innovation*. Baltimore, MD: Johns Hopkins University Press.

Limbo, Rana, Debra Brandon, Denise Côté-Arsenault, Karen Kavanaugh, Amy Kuebelbeck, and Charlotte Wool. 2017. "Perinatal Palliative Care as an Essential Element of Childbearing Choices." *Nursing Outlook* 65 (1): 123–5.

Lu, Mathew. 2011. "Abortion and Virtue Ethics." In *Persons, Moral Worth, and Embryos: A Critical Analysis of Pro-Choice Arguments*, edited by Stephen Napier, 101–23. New York: Springer.

MacIntyre, Alasdair C. 1999. *Dependent Rational Animals: Why Human Beings Need the Virtues*. Chicago, IL: Open Court.

McCaffrey, Martin J. 2016. "Trisomy 13 and 18: Selecting the Road Previously Not Taken." *American Journal of Medical Genetics Part C: Seminars in Medical Genetics* 172 (3): 251–6.

Meadow, William and John Lantos. 2009. "Moral Reflections on Neonatal Intensive Care." *Pediatrics* 123 (2): 595–7.

Meadow, William, Joanne Lagatta, Bree Andrews, and John Lantos. 2012b. "The Mathematics of Morality for Neonatal Resuscitation." *Clinics in Perinatology* 39 (4): 941–56.

Meadow, William, Sally Cohen-Cutler, Bridget Spelke, Anna Kim, Melissa Plesac, Kirsten Weis, and Joanne Lagatta. 2012a. "The Prediction and Cost of Futility in the NICU." *Acta Paediatrica* 101 (4): 397–402.

Muraskas, Jonathan and Kayhan Parsi. 2008. "The Cost of Saving the Tiniest Lives: NICUs Versus Prevention." *Virtual Mentor* 10 (10): 655–8.

Reinders, Hans J. 2000. *The Future of the Disabled in Liberal Society*. Notre Dame: University of Notre Dame Press.

Saigal, Saroj, Barbara L. Stoskopf, David Feeny, William Furlong, Elizabeth Burrows, Peter L. Rosenbaum, and Lorraine Hoult. 1999. "Differences in Preferences for Neonatal Outcomes among Health Care Professionals, Parents, and Adolescents." *Journal of the American Medical Association* 281 (21): 1991–7.

Sandelowski, Margarete and Linda Corson Jones. 1996. "'Healing Fictions': Stories of Choosing in the Aftermath of the Detection of Fetal Anomalies." *Social Science & Medicine* 42 (3): 353–61.

Sandelowski, Margarete and Julie Barroso. 2005. "The Travesty of Choosing after Positive Prenatal Diagnosis." *Journal of Obstetric, Gynecologic, & Neonatal Nursing* 34: 307–18.

Sullivan, Nora and Eoghan de Faoite. 2017. "Psychological Impact of Abortion due to Fetal Anomaly: A Review of Published Research." *Issues in Law & Medicine* 32 (1): 19–30.

Watt, Helen. 2017. "Abortion for Life-Limiting Foetal Anomaly: Beneficial When and For Whom?" *Clinical Ethics* 12 (1): 1–10.

Williams-Reade, Jackie, Angela L. Lamson, Sharon M. Knight, Mark B. White, Sharon M. Ballard, and Priti P. Desai. 2015. "The Clinical, Operational, and Financial Worlds of Neonatal Palliative Care: A Focused Ethnography." *Palliative & Supportive Care* 13 (2): 179–86.

Wool, Charlotte and Martha Dudek. 2013. "Exploring the Perceptions and the Role of Genetic Counselors in the Emerging Field of Perinatal Palliative Care." *Journal of Genetic Counseling* 22 (4): 533–43.

Wool, Charlotte, Denise Côté-Arsenault, Beth Perry Black, Erin Denney-Koelsch, Sujeong Kim, and Karen Kavanaugh. 2016. "Provision of Services in Perinatal Palliative Care: A Multicenter Survey in the United States." *Journal of Palliative Medicine* 19 (3): 279–85.

Wool, Charlotte, Rana Limbo, and Erin M. Denney-Koelsch. 2018. "'I Would Do It All Over Again': Cherishing Time and the Absence of Regret in Continuing a Pregnancy after a Life-Limiting Diagnosis." *The Journal of Clinical Ethics* 29 (3): 227–36.

Wool, Charlotte. 2013. "Clinician Confidence and Comfort in Providing Perinatal Palliative Care." *Journal of Obstetric, Gynecologic & Neonatal Nursing* 42 (1): 48–58.

Wool, Charlotte. 2015. "Clinician Perspectives of Barriers in Perinatal Palliative Care." *MCN: The American Journal of Maternal/Child Nursing* 40 (10): 44–50.

Index

Printed in the United States
by Baker & Taylor Publisher Services